Nanotechnology for Cancer Therapy

ABOUT THE BOOK

Nanotechnology offers the unprecedented and paradigm-changing opportunity to study and interact with normal and cancer cells in real time, at the molecular and cellular scales, and during the earliest stages of the cancer process. Through the concerted development of nanoscale devices or devices with nanoscale materials and components, the NCI Alliance for Nanotechnology in Cancer will facilitate in near future their integration within the existing cancer research infrastructure. Nanotechnology is manipulating matter at nanometer level and the application of the same to medicine is called nanomedicine. Nanotechnology holds promise for advanced diagnostics, targeted drug delivery, and biosensors. In the long-term, medical nanorobots will allow instant pathogen diagnosis and extermination, individual cell surgery in vivo, and improvement of natural physiological function. Nanotechnology is expected to have a dramatic impact on medicine. The application of nanotechnology for treatment, diagnosis, monitoring, and control of biological systems is now often referred to as nanomedicine. Among many possible applications of nanotechnology in medicine, the use of various nanomaterials as pharmaceutical delivery systems for drugs, DNA, and imaging agents has gained increasing attention. Many varieties of nanoparticles are available, such as different polymeric and metal nanoparticles, liposomes, niosomes, solid lipid particles, micelles, quantum dots, dendrimers, microcapsules, cells, cell ghosts, lipoproteins, and different nanoassemblies. The book will serve as an ultimate resource book for everyone who would like to know the wide range of prospects in the emerging applications of Nanotechnology for Cancer Therapy.

ABOUT THE AUTHOR

Mahesh Narayan, received his master's degree in Biotechnology from University of Leeds, U.K, in Molecular Biology and Genetics, where he is currently working as research fellow. His scope of interest is Genomic and Phenotypic Evolution of Tumor Cells under Chemotherapeutic Stresses and Viro-immunological approaches as an alternative perspective in Cancer Therapy. He has received various awards viz. DBT-research Associateship, young scientist by ISGBRD; ICAR, recognition award for research.

Nanotechnology for CANCER THERAPY

Mahesh Narayan

AMIGA PRESS. INC
Delhi -110051

AMIGA PRESS INC.
H.O :- 28-A, Indra Park,
Chander Nagar, Delhi :- 110051 (India)
Tel :- 011-22504028, +91-98736-57000
Email :- amigapress@gmail.com
amigaeditorial@gmail.com
amigapub@gmail.com
Website :- www.amigapress.co.in

This edition is published by Amiga Press Inc.

ISBN : 978-93-87295-41-4

First Published 2019

Printed and bound by Replika Press Pvt. Ltd.

Preface

Cancer nanotechnology is currently under intense development for applications in cancer imaging, molecular diagnosis and targeted therapy. The basic rationale is that nanometer-sized particles, such as biodegradable micelles, semiconductor quantum dots and iron oxide nanocrystals, have functional or structural properties that are not available from either molecular or macroscopic agents. When linked with biotargeting ligands, such as monoclonal antibodies, peptides or small molecules, these nanoparticles are used to target malignant tumors with high affinity and specificity. In the 'mesoscopic' size range of 5-100 nm in diameter, nanoparticles also have large surface areas and functional groups for conjugating to multiple diagnostic (e.g., optical, radioisotopic or magnetic) and therapeutic (e.g., anticancer) agents. Recent advances have led to multifunctional nanoparticle probes for molecular and cellular imaging, nanoparticle drugs for targeted therapy, and integrated nanodevices for early cancer detection and screening. These developments have opened exciting opportunities for personalized oncology in which cancer detection, diagnosis and therapy are tailored to each individual's molecular profile, and also for predictive oncology, in which genetic/molecular information is used to predict tumor development, progression and clinical outcome.

Nanotechnology may also be useful for developing ways to eradicate cancer cells without harming healthy, neighboring cells. Scientists hope to use nanotechnology to create therapeutic agents that target specific cells and deliver the toxin in a controlled, time-release manner. Researchers aim eventually to create single agents that are able to both detect cancer and deliver treatment. The ultimate goal of this research is nanoparticles that will circulate through the body, detect cancer-associated molecular changes, assist with imaging, release a therapeutic agent, and then monitor the effectiveness of the intervention.

Enormous progress is being made in understanding the molecular basis of endocrine-related cancer, and this brings great potential to design improved therapeutic strategies. Although the pharmaceutical industry prefers to develop small-molecule anticancer agents that can be administered to patients orally (very convenient to use), macro-molecular drugs and delivery systems, including antibodies, proteins and polymer conjugates, are establishing their niche in modern chemotherapy. It is now universally agreed that combination approaches, perhaps involving small molecules (endocrine and chemotherapy), macromolecular drugs such as antibodies, and DDS, including polymer therapeutics, will probably be required to increase therapeutic index and circumvent all routes to resistance.

Drug delivery techniques were established to deliver or control the amount, rate and, sometimes location of a drug in the body to optimize its therapeutic effect, convenience and dose. Combining a well established drug formulation with a new delivery system is a relatively low risk activity and can be used to enhance a company's product portfolio by extending the drug's commercial life-cycle. Although not exhausting, this is a representative selection reflecting current industrial trends. Most companies are developing pharmaceutical applications, mainly for drug delivery. Most major and established pharmaceutical companies have internal research programs on drug delivery that are on formulations or dispersions containing components down to nano sizes. With the total global investment in nanotechnologies currently at 5 billion, the global market is estimated to reach over 1 trillion by 2011-2015. Nano and Micro technologies are part of the latest advanced solutions and new paradigm for decreasing the discovery and development time for new drugs and potentially reducing the development costs.

Nanotechnology has tremendous potential to make an important contribution in cancer prevention, detection, diagnosis, imaging and treatment. It can target a tumor, carry imaging capability to document the presence of tumor, sense pathophysiological defects in tumor cells, deliver therapeutic genes or drugs based on tumor characteristics, respond to external triggers to release the agent and document the tumor response and identify residual tumor cells. Nanoparticles are important because of their nanoscaled structure but nanoparticles in cancer are still bigger than many anticancer drugs.

This is a reference book. All the matter is just compiled and edited in nature, taken from the various sources which are in public domain.

The book will serve as an ultimate resource book for everyone who would like to know the wide range of prospects in the emerging applications of Nanotechnology for Cancer Therapy.

—*Editor*

Contents

1

Cancer Treatment by Nanotechnology

Nanotechnology may also be useful for developing ways to eradicate cancer cells without harming healthy, neighboring cells. Scientists hope to use nanotechnology to create therapeutic agents that target specific cells and deliver the toxin in a controlled, time-release manner. Researchers aim eventually to create single agents that are able to both detect cancer and deliver treatment. The ultimate goal of this research is nanoparticles that will circulate through the body, detect cancer-associated molecular changes, assist with imaging, release a therapeutic agent, and then monitor the effectiveness of the intervention.

TOOLS FOR THE TREATMENT

Research is being done on a number of nanoparticles that will facilitate drug delivery. One such molecule with potential to link treatment with detection and diagnosis is known as a dendrimer. A useful feature of dendrimers is their branching shape, which gives them vast amounts of surface area to which scientists can attach therapeutic agents or other biologically active molecules.

A single dendrimer can carry a molecule that recognizes cancer cells, a therapeutic agent to kill those cells, and a molecule that recognizes the signals of cell death. Researchers hope to manipulate dendrimers to release their contents only in the presence of certain trigger molecules associated with cancer. Following drug release, the dendrimers may also report back whether they are successfully killing their targets.

Nanoshells, another recent invention, are miniscule beads coated with gold. By manipulating the thickness of the layers making up the nanoshells, scientists can design these beads to absorb specific wavelengths of light. The most useful nanoshells are those that absorb near-infrared light, which can easily penetrate several centimeters of human tissue. The absorption of light by the nanoshells creates an intense heat that is lethal to cells. Researchers can already link nanoshells to antibodies that recognize cancer cells. Scientists envision letting these nanoshells seek out their cancerous targets, then applying near-infrared light. In laboratory cultures, the heat generated by the light-absorbing nanoshells has successfully killed tumor cells while leaving neighboring cells intact.

Use of Nanotechnologies in Patient Care

These technologies are in various stages of discovery and development. Experts believe that quantum dots, nanopores and other devices for detection and diagnosis may be available for clinical use in five to 15 years. Therapeutic agents are expected to be available within a similar time frame. Devices that integrate detection and therapy could be used clinically in about 15 or 20 years.

Nanotechnology has the potential to have a revolutionary impact on cancer diagnosis and therapy. It is universally accepted that early detection of cancer is essential even before anatomic anomalies are visible. A major challenge in cancer diagnosis in the 21st century is to be able to determine the exact relationship between cancer biomarkers and the clinical pathology, as well as, to be able to non-invasively detect tumors at an early stage for maximum therapeutic benefit. For breast cancer, for instance, the goal of molecular imaging is to be able to accurately diagnose when the tumor mass has approximately 100-1000 cells, as opposed to the current techniques like mammography, which require more than a million cells for accurate clinical diagnosis.

In cancer therapy, targeting and localized delivery are the key challenges. To wage an effective war against cancer, we have to have the ability to selectively attack the cancer cells, while saving the normal tissue from excessive burdens of drug toxicity. However, because many anticancer drugs are designed to simply kill cancer cells, often in a semi-specific fashion, the distribution of anticancer drugs in healthy organs or tissues is especially undesirable due to the potential for severe side effects. Consequently, systemic application of these drugs often causes severe side effects in other tissues (e.g. bone marrow suppression, cardiomyopathy, neurotoxicity), which greatly limits the maximal allowable dose of the drug.

In addition, rapid elimination and widespread distribution into non-targeted organs and tissues requires the administration of a drug in large quantities, which is often not economical and sometimes complicated due to non-specific toxicity. This vicious cycle of large doses and the concurrent toxicity is a major limitation of current cancer therapy. In many instances, it has been observed that the patient succumbs to the ill effects of the drug toxicity far earlier than the tumor burden. Nanotechnolgy still needs to improve in the following major areas.

- Science and technologies for cancer diagnostic and imaging techniques using nanoparticles as reporter platforms and contrast enhancing agents;
- Bionalaytical nanotechnology for detection of biomarkers
- Nanoparticle platforms polymeric nanoparticles, lipid nanoparticles, metal nanoparticles, magnetic nanoparticles, and self-assembling nanosystems;
- Synthetic chemistry required to design and optimize new strategies for nanoparticle preparation and functionalization;
- Therapeutic targeted and intra-cellular drug and gene delivery using nanocarriers;
- Nanoparticles for delivery of electromagnetic energy for hyperthermia and thermal ablation of tumors;
- Theoretical modeling of nanoparticle processes in biological and medical environments, and of drug and gene delivery;
- Combination therapies (drug and energy delivery) using nanoparticles
- Clinical diagnosis and therapy of prostate, breast, and liver cancer.

CHALLENGES RELATED WITH NANOTECHNOLOGY

Today, much of the science on the nanoscale is basic research, designed to reach a better understanding of how matter behaves on this small scale. Matter behaves differently on the nanoscale than it does at larger levels. The factors that govern larger systems do not necessarily apply on the nanoscale. Because nanomaterials have large surface areas relative to their volumes, phenomena like friction and sticking are more important than they are in larger systems. These factors will affect use both inside and outside the body.

Other challenges apply specifically to the use of nanostructures within biological systems. Nanostructures can be so small that the body may clear them too rapidly for them to be effective in detection or imaging. Larger nanoparticles may accumulate in vital organs, creating a toxicity problem. Scientists will need to consider these factors as they anticipate how nanostructures will behave in the human body and attempt to create devices the body will accept.

Creation of Nanodevices

There are two basic approaches for creating nanodevices. Scientists refer to these methods as the top-down approach and the bottom-up approach. The top-down approach involves molding or etching materials into smaller components. This approach has traditionally been used in making parts for computers and electronics. The bottom-up approach involves assembling structures atom-by-atom or molecule-by-molecule and may prove useful in manufacturing devices used in medicine.

Advantages of to Biological Systems

Most animal cells are 10,000 to 20,000 nanometers in diameter. This means that nanoscale devices (having at least one dimension less than 100 nanometers) can enter cells and the organelles inside them to interact with DNA and proteins.

Tools developed through nanotechnology may be able to detect disease in a very small amount of cells or tissue. They may also be able to enter and monitor cells within a living body. Miniaturization will allow the tools for many different tests to be situated together on the same small device.

This means that nanotechnology could make it possible to run many diagnostic tests simultaneously as well as with more sensitivity. In general, nanotechnology may offer a faster and more efficient means for scientists to do much of what they do now.

Cancer Detection and Diagnosis

Detection of cancer at an early stage is a critical step in improving cancer treatment. Currently, detection and diagnosis of cancer usually depend on changes in cells and tissues that are detected by a doctor's physical exam or imaging expertise. Instead, scientists would like to make it possible to detect cancer when the earliest molecular changes are present, long before a physical exam or imaging technology is effective. To do this, they need a new set of tools. Nanotechnology is uniquely promising as an early detection tool for several reasons:

To successfully detect cancer at its earliest stages, scientists must be able to detect molecular changes even when they occur only in a small percentage of cells. This means the necessary tools must be extremely sensitive. The potential for nanostructures to enter and analyze single cells suggests they could meet this need. Many nanotechnology tools will make it possible for clinicians to run tests without physically altering the cells or tissue they take from a patient. This is important because the samples clinicians use to screen for cancer are often in limited supply. Scientists would like to perform tests without altering cells, so they can be used again if further tests are needed.

Reductions in the size of tools means that many tests can be run on a single small device. This will make screening faster and more cost-efficient.

Tools for Early Detection

The cantilevel is one tool with potential to aid in cancer diagnosis. Nanoscale cantilevers-tiny bars anchored at one end-can be engineered to bind to molecules associated with cancer. They may bind to altered DNA sequences or proteins that are present in certain types of cancer. When the cancer-associated molecules bind to the cantilevers, changes in surface tension cause the cantilevers to bend. By monitoring whether or not the cantilevers are bent, scientists can tell whether the cancer molecules are present. Scientists hope this bending will be evident even when the altered molecules are present in very low concentrations. This will be useful in detecting early molecular events in the development of cancer.

Other technologies will focus on improved methods of reading the genetic code on single strands of DNA to detect errors that may contribute to cancer. Scientists believe nanopores, tiny holes that allow DNA to pass through one strand at a time, will make DNA sequencing more efficient. As DNA passes through a nanopore, scientists can monitor the shape and electrical properties of each base on the strand. Because these properties are unique for each of the four bases that make up the genetic code, scientists can use the passage of DNA through a nanopore to decipher the encoded information, including errors in the code known to be associated with cancer.

Even smaller than nanopores are nanotubes. Nanotubes, carbon rods about half the diameter of a molecule of DNA, will also help identify DNA changes associated with cancer. Beyond detecting the presence of altered genes, these materials may help researchers pinpoint the exact location of those changes. Mutated regions associated with cancer are first tagged with bulky molecules. Using a nanotube tip resembling the needle on a record player, researchers can then trace the physical shape of DNA. A computer translates this information into a topographical map. The bulky molecules identify the regions on the map where mutations are present. Since the location of mutations can influence the effects they have on a cell, these techniques will be important in predicting disease.

Researchers would like to be able to detect the early signs or precursors of cancer in cells without removing them from the body. One tool that will allow scientists to detect critical changes in DNA in the body is quantum dots. Quantum dots are tiny crystals that glow when they are stimulated by ultraviolet light. The wavelength, or color, of the light depends on the size of the crystal. Latex beads filled with these crystals can be designed to bind to specific DNA sequences. When the crystals are stimulated by light, the colors they emit act as dyes that light up the sequences of interest. By combining different sized quantum dots within a single bead, scientists can create probes that release a distinct spectrum of various colors and intensities of lights, serving as a sort of spectral bar code.

To detect cancer, scientists can design beads containing quantum dots to bind to sequences of DNA that are associated with cancer. When the quantum dots are stimulated with light, they will emit their unique bar codes, or labels, making the critical, cancer-associated DNA sequences visible. The vast number of possible combinations of quantum dots means that scientists can create many unique labels, which can be used at the same time. This will allow scientists to look simultaneously at numerous regions of DNA. This will be important in the detection of cancer, which results from many different changes within a cell.

TYPES OF NANOTECHNOLOGY

Nanotechnology is the science and creation of materials at a molecular level. Nanotechnology applications are used in medicine, chemistry, the environment, energy companies, and communication. Whether it is through nanotechnology education or nanotechnology application, this science continues to evolve and find more uses in everyday life. The use of nanotechnologies in medicine has provided many medical breakthroughs. Some of the medical nanotechnology applications are for diagnostics. These are used to assist in identifying DNA and helping detect genetic sequences.

Other uses of nanotechnology in medicine are in drug delivery and tissue engineering. Drug delivery can help in cancer treatments by administering drugs via implant versus the traditional injections. Tissue engineering is a new nanotechnology and involves repairing or artificially reproducing damaged tissue. Using molecular nanotechnology in chemistry and the environment has already resulted in positive benefits. Chemical catalysis is a process of reducing pollutants using a reagent or catalyst. This can be especially helpful if used in vehicle fuel cells or catalytic converters to reduce car emissions. Filtration is another one of the nanotechnology applications that can help the environment. Extremely small holes in the filtration, known as nanofiltration, remove ions for wastewater treatment or air purification. Slightly larger holes are used in a type of filtration called ultra filtration and its current application is for renal dialysis.

Now that nanotechnology has been in the public eye for twenty years, and well-funded for half a decade, it's worth a quick look at just what it is—and how it got that way. When the word "nanotechnology" was introduced to the public by Eric Drexler's 1986 book *Engines of Creation*, it meant something very specific: small precise machines built out of molecules, which could build more molecular machines and products—large, high-performance products. This goal or aspect of nanotechnology now goes by several names, including molecular nanotechnology, molecular manufacturing, and productive nanosystems. The reason for this renaming is that "nanotechnology" has become a broad and inclusive term, but it's still important to distinguish molecular manufacturing from all the other types. I'll talk about molecular manufacturing, and why it is unique and important, after surveying some of the other types of nanotechnology.

With the funding of the U.S. National Nanotechnology Initiative (NNI), there has been a strong financial incentive to define nanotechnology so that one's own research counts—but not so broadly that everyone's research counts. There has been a less focused, but still real, incentive to define the goals of nanotechnology aggressively, to justify major funding, but not too aggressively, lest it sound scary or implausible.

With all the different research fields applying the above rules to a wide variety of research, it is not surprising that there's no single hard-edged definition of nanotechnology that everyone can agree on. Perhaps the most commonly quoted definition of nanotechnology is the one used by the NNI: "Nanotechnology is the understanding and control of matter at dimensions of roughly 1 to 100 nanometers, where unique phenomena enable novel applications." I don't know how they decided on the size scale; thinking cynically, it might have had something to do with the fact that computer chips were just about to gain features smaller than 100 nanometers, so they were guaranteed at least one early success.

Nanotechnology can be even broader than that. A rough rule of thumb is: if it's too small to see with an ordinary light microscope, it's likely to be considered nanotechnology. Without using special physics tricks, light can't be used to see anything smaller than half a wavelength of light, which is a few hundred nanometers. Because some optics technology uses structures smaller than light (such as photonic crystals) to manipulate light, you will sometimes see optics researchers describe their work as nanotechnology. However, because these structures tend to be larger than the official 100-nm cutoff, many nanotechnologists will reject this usage. Another point of contention is how unique the "unique phenomena enabl[ing] novel applications" have to be. For example, some nanotechnology simply uses ordinary materials like clay, in smaller chunks, in fairly ordinary ways. They can get new material properties; they are using nanoscale materials; they are studying them with new techniques; but is it really nanotechnology, or is it just materials science? It might as well be called nanotech, seems to be the consensus. It's providing early successes for the field and it's putting "nano" into consumers' hands in a beneficial, non-threatening way.

Another kind of nanotechnology involves building increasingly large and intricate molecules. Some of these molecules can be very useful: for example, it appears possible to combine a cancer-cell-recognizer, a toxic drug, and a component that shows up in MRI scans, into a single molecule that kills cancer cells while showing you where they were and leaving the rest of the body untouched. This is a little bit different from traditional chemistry in that the chemist isn't trying to create a new molecule with a single function, but rather to join together several different functions into one connected package.

Some new nanomaterials have genuinely new properties. For example, small mineral particles can be transparent to visible light, which makes them useful in sunscreen. Even smaller particles can glow in useful colors, forming more-stable markers for biomedical research. For related reasons, small particles can be useful additions to computer circuits, lending their quantum effects to make smaller and better transistors.

We should talk about semiconductors (computer chips), a major application of nanotechnology. Feature sizes on mainstream silicon chips are well below 100 nanometers now. This obviously is a great success for nanotechnology (as defined by the NNI). From one point of view, semiconductor makers are continuing to do what they have always done: make chips smaller and faster using silicon-based transistors. From another point of view, as sizes shrink, their task is rapidly getting harder, and they are inventing new technology every day just to keep up with expectations. There are more unusual computer-chip designs underway as well, most of which use nanotechnology of one form or another, from quantum-dot transistors to sub-wavelength optics (plasmonics) to holographic storage to buckytube-based mechanical switches. Which brings us to buckytubes. Buckytubes are remarkable molecules that were discovered not long ago. They are tiny strips of graphite, rolled up with the sides fastened together to form a seamless tube. They are very strong, very stiff, and can be quite long in proportion to their width; four-centimeter long buckytubes have been reported, which is more than ten million times the width of the tube. Some buckytubes are world-class conductors and electron emitters. They may be useful in a wide variety of applications.

And what about those quantum effects? According to the NNI, "At the nanoscale, the physical, chemical, and biological properties of materials differ in fundamental and valuable ways from the properties of individual atoms and molecules or bulk matter." Materials are of course made up of atoms, which contain electrons, and it is the interaction of electrons that gives materials most of their properties. In very small chunks of material, the electrons interact differently, which can create new material properties. Nanoparticles can be more chemically active; as mentioned above, they can fluoresce; they can even participate in weird physics such as quantum computers. But, as the above overview should make clear, a lot of "nanotechnology" does not make use of these quantum effects.

Molecular manufacturing (MM) is a fairly mundane branch of nanotech, or it would be if not for the political controversy that has swirled around it. The idea is simple: Use nanoscale machines as construction tools, joining molecular fragments into more machines. Every biological cell contains molecular machines that do exactly that. There are, however, a few reasons why molecular manufacturing has been highly controversial.

Much of the controversy stems from the fact that MM proposes to use engineered devices to build duplicate devices. Although biology can do this, intuition suggests that such self-duplication requires some special spark of complexity or something even more numinous: surely a simple engineered machine can't be so lifelike! This ultimate spark of vitalism is fading as we learn how machinelike cellular molecules actually are, and as increasingly detailed plans make it clear that hardware does not have to be very complex in order to make duplicate hardware. (Even the software doesn't have to be very complex, just intricate and well-designed. This has been known by computer scientists for many decades, but the paradigm has taken a while to shift in the wider world.)

There is another problem with self-replication: in some forms, it may be dangerous. In 1986, Eric Drexler warned that tiny engineered self-replicators could outcompete natural life, turning the biosphere into boring copies of themselves: "grey goo." This formed a cornerstone of Bill Joy's essay "Why

The Future Doesn't Need Us," which hit just as the NNI was ramping up. No nanoscientist wanted to be associated with a poorly-understood technology that might destroy the world, and the easiest thing was to assert that MM was simply impossible. (Modern MM designs do not use small self-replicators; in fact, they have been obsolete since Drexler's 1992 technical book *Nanosystems*.)

A third source of controversy is that MM plans to use diamond as its major building material, not bio-based polymers like protein and DNA. (Some pathways to this capability, including the pathway favored by Drexler, go through a biopolymer stage.) Although there is a wide variety of reactions that can form diamond and graphite, living organisms do not build with these materials, so there is no existence proof that such structures can be built using point-by-point computer-controlled molecular deposition. If diamond-like structures can be built by molecular manufacturing techniques, they should have astonishingly high performance characteristics. To those who study MM, its projected high performance indicates that researchers should work toward this goal with a focused intensity not seen since the Manhattan Project. To those who have not studied MM, talk of motors a million times more powerful than today's merely seems fanciful, a reason (or an excuse) to discount the entire field.

At least as problematic as the extreme technical claims are the concerns about the extreme implications of molecular manufacturing. It is rare that a technology comes along which revolutionizes society in a decade or so, and even more rare that such things are correctly predicted in advance. It is very tempting to dismiss claims of unstable arms races, wholesale destruction of existing jobs, and widespread personal capacity for mass destruction, as improbable.

However, all the skepticism in the world won't change the laws of physics. In more than two decades (almost five, if you count from Richard Feynman's visionary speech), no one has found a reason why MM, even diamond-based MM, shouldn't work. In fact, the more work that's done, the less complex it appears. Predicting social responses to technology is even more difficult than predicting technology itself, but it seems beyond plausibility that such a powerful capability won't have at least some disruptive effects—perhaps fatally disruptive, unless we can understand the potential and find ways to bypass the worst pitfalls.

In the near future, nanotechnology in the broad sense will continue to develop dozens of interesting technologies and capabilities, leading to hundreds of improved capabilities and applications. Meanwhile, molecular manufacturing will continue to move closer, despite the (rapidly fading) opposition to the idea. Sometime in the next few years, someone will have the vision to fund a targeted study of molecular manufacturing's potential; less than a decade after that, general-purpose nanoscale manufacturing will be a reality that the world will have to deal with. Molecular manufacturing will build virtually unlimited quantities of new products as rapidly as the software can be designed—and it should be noted that most of today's physical products are far less complex than today's software. Molecular manufacturing will both enable and eclipse large areas of nanotechnology, further accelerating the achievements of the field. We are in for some interesting times.

GOLD NANOPARTICLES SHOWING POTENTIAL FOR NONINVASIVE CANCER TREATMENT

A father-and-son team of researchers from the University of California, San Francisco, and Georgia Institute of Technology have shown that targeted gold nanoparticles combined with a subsequent laser ablation can kill oral cancer cells. Building on their previous work that used gold nanoparticles to detect cancer, the investigators now are heating the particles and using them as agents to destroy malignant cells. Their study findings are reported in the journal Cancer Letters. "In an earlier study we showed how gold nanoparticles could be bound to malignant cells, making cancer detection easier. Now we have examined how the particles' ability to absorb light helps kill those cancer cells," said principal author Ivan El-Sayed, M.D., of the UCSF Medical Center.

Many cancer cells have a protein, known as epidermal growth factor receptor (EGFR), distributed widely on the outside of their cell membranes. In contrast, healthy cells typically do not produce much of this protein. By attaching gold nanoparticles to an antibody for EGFR (anti-EGFR), the researchers were able to get the nanoparticles to specifically attach themselves to the cancer cells.

In the new study, the researchers incubated two oral squamous carcinoma cell lines and one benign epithelial cell line with anti-EFGR conjugated gold nanoparticles and then exposed them to continuous visible light from an argon laser. "The malignant cells required less than half the laser energy to be killed than the benign cells," said Ivan El-Sayed. "In addition, we observed no photothermal destruction of any type of cell in the absence of gold nanoparticles at these low laser powers."

When combined with the researchers' earlier work using the same nanoparticles to detect oral carcinoma, this research points the way to a multifunctional nanoparticle for detecting and treating oral cancer. "We now have the potential to design an 'all in one' active agent that can be used to noninvasively find the cancer and then kill it," added Ivan El-Sayed. "This holds great promise for a number of types of cancer."

This work is detailed in a paper titled, "Selective laser photo-thermal therapy of epithelial carcinoma using anti-EGFR antibody conjugated gold nanoparticles." Recent successful medical trials of a cancer treatment involving the use of "nanotechnology" may open up important new avenues for the diagnosis and treatment of other cancers and diseases.

Nanotechnology is a broad term covering the building of structures and "machines" on an atomic or molecular scale-in the range from 1 to 100 nanometres. A nanometre is one billionth of a metre or about the size of 10 hydrogen atoms. The techniques range from various chemical and biological processes used to "construct" structures-in some cases atom by atom-to the etching methods used to produce computer chips.

The field of nanotechnology has over the last decade or so been surrounded by considerable hype. Some of the visions of what is possible in medicine conjure up the Science Fiction classic film Fantastic Voyage where tiny submarine ships were injected into the body and travelled through the bloodstream to eradicate foreign bodies. The reality is more prosaic, but the potential is nonetheless exciting.

Many of the standard radiation and drug therapies now used to treat cancers can have serious side effects. The use of radiation and chemicals to kill fast-growing tumour cells inevitably affects and kills other cells in the body. Nanotechnology offers the possibility of far more precisely localising the treatment and thus minimising the damage to healthy tissue.

In early April, the nanotechnology company pSivida announced the very promising results of the Phase 2 clinical trials of its product "BrachySil" for patients with liver cancer.

BrachySil is a tiny structure about one-millionth of a metre in size and made up of modified particles of silicon impregnated with the radioactive isotope of phosphorus 32P. Unlike other radiation treatments that involve focussing beams of radiation on tumours, BrachySil is injected directly into the cancer using a fine gauge needle. By using 32P, the radiation is limited to a range of just 8 millimetres, resulting in the killing of tumour cells rather than healthy tissue.

For several years, doctors have been using a similar technique known as brachytherapy-injecting radioisotopes directly into tumours. The difficulty was that the injected material would not remain in the cancer, but would over time be carried to other parts of the body. The advantage of BrachySil is that its silicon structures, while small, prevent the radioisotope from leaking away.

The result is that the dose of radiation is focussed very precisely on the tumour itself. The silicon eventually breaks down and is excreted. 32P, which has a half-life of 14 days, eventually decomposes to stable isotopes or is excreted. Because the treatment is localised, the side effects are likely to be less than other forms of brachytherapy. None have been observed to date, although the long-term impact of the treatment is not known.

BrachySil consists of tiny pockets made up of silicon microparticles. The pores or holes in the silicon pocket are the size of about 10 atoms. Radioactive phosphorus is bombarded into the structure. Because of its method of delivery of radiation doses, the treatment may well be applicable to a broader range of cancers than other forms of brachytherapy, which is currently limited to prostate and liver cancers.

The clinical trial of BrachySil was undertaken at the Singapore General Hospital beginning in mid-2004. It involved eight patients suffering from primary liver cancer (where the tumours have not spread to a secondary site). They were given CT scans before and after the injection of BrachySil to determine the impact on the tumours and were monitored for possible side effects.

After 12 weeks of the treatment, smaller tumours were completely eradicated. The most extraordinary finding, however, was that all tumours were reduced by an average of 80 percent-a result not seen in other treatments. After the trial results were announced, the company received a flood of inquiries and was forced to announce on its website that testing was still in its early stages.

Worldwide, liver cancer is not one of the most prevalent cancers. Nevertheless, more than half a million new cases are diagnosed every year-some 45 percent of them in China. Causes of liver cancer include infection by parasites such as the Chinese liver fluke. Liver cancer can also be related to hepatitis, exposure to radiation and to the irritant Polyvinyl Chloride.

OTHER APPLICATIONS

An article published in the British scientific journal Nature in March entitled "Cancer Nanotechnology: Opportunities and Challenges" provided an overview of the diverse array of nanodevices and their possible application. These included "nanovectors" to provide the targetted delivery of anticancer drugs as well as "nanowires" and "nanocantilever arrays" for the early detection of pre-cancerous and malignant lesions.

Many of the devices are still in the process of development, but some are being used or, like BrachySil, are in the testing process. The earliest known application was the use of "liposomes" or small spheres that have been used to treat cancers such as Kaposi's sarcoma for about 10 years. They are now being used in cases of breast cancer and ovarian cancer.

"Nanovectors" are generally made up of three basic parts: a core; the contents which may be a specific drug or chemical used for imaging; and a surface coating. The coating is needed both to target cancerous tissue and to prevent the body's own defence mechanisms from engulfing and destroying the nanovector.

In 2003, US scientists developed a "nanoshell" made up of a silica core and a thin gold metal shell modified to strongly absorb near-infrared (NIR) light. The nanoshells were injected into mice, which were then exposed to a safe dose of NIR radiation causing cancer cells to die. Magnetic Resonance Imaging (MRI) scans enabled the scientists to monitor exactly where the nanospheres were located and thus successfully target cancer cells.

Scientists have also built nanoshells to deliver small precise doses of drugs to tumours. It is hoped that such techniques will be able to avoid many of the serious side effects that are associated with current chemotherapy.

At the end of March, scientists at the Institute of Bio-engineering and Nanotechnology in Singapore published their findings on the use of polymer nanoparticles to deliver anti-cancer drugs directly to diseased tissue. The results showed that the technique applied to mice was effective in conveying the drug doxorubicin to breast tumours. The scientists hope that clinical trials will follow in the next five years. The nanoparticles were tagged with biological signals to enable them to hone in on the cancer cells. This was achieved by modifying the particles to be sensitive to both temperature and pH. The tumour cells, which are characteristically slightly acidic, caused the nanosphere to "deform" and release the drugs at the exact site of the cancer cells. The outer shell was also coated with bioactive compounds to protect the particle from degradation and digestive fluids.

Nanoparticles have also been modified to provide better cancer detection. Researchers at Washington University School of Medicine demonstrated that very small human melanoma tumours growing in mice-that are not discernible using a direct MRI scan-would "light up" and be easily located some 30 minutes after the mice were injected with specialised nanoparticles.

Stanford University nanotechnology expert Stephen Quake has predicted within a decade that the diagnosis and treatment of cancers and other diseases will be "carried out automatically, in a few seconds or minutes, on a just a handful of cells or their contents". While the prediction may turn out to be overly optimistic, there is no doubt that nanotechnology may well open the way for a new generation of cancer treatments that are more effective and less damaging than those currently available.

CUTTING SIDE EFFECTS

Scientists say they have developed a way to deliver lethal drug doses to tumours without causing side-effects, such as nausea and hair loss.

The Australian team has used nanotechnology to create tiny particles which specifically attack cancer cells, but leave healthy tissue unaffected.

The particles-or mini-cells-are tagged with anti-cancer antibodies so they zero in on their target.

The research features in the journal Cancer Cell.

It is hoped the technique could treat tumours in the breast, ovaries, colon and lungs.

So far it has been used in mice and dogs, and the researchers plan to begin human trials shortly.

Traditional chemotherapy typically involves subjecting the patient's entire body to powerful drugs, which can cause a range of severe side-effects.

Bacteria Cells

The mini-cells-about one-fifth the size of a normal cell-were created from bacteria cells stripped of their reproductive powers.

They were then loaded with cancer drugs, and tagged with antibodies which are attracted to cancerous tumours.

Once the cell reaches the cancer, the drug is released directly into the malignant growth.

Researcher Jennifer MacDiarmid, from Sydney-based biotechnology company EnGeneIC, said: "There is no other system where you can get so much drug concentrated into a little parcel."

In tests, the technique reduced tumours in animals without side effects-and by using only a very small amount of drug.

Dr MacDiarmid said the treatment could potentially be used on any solid tumours.

She said the technique potentially paved the way for customised drug cocktails for individual patients. Professor Quentin Pankhurst, of the London Centre for Nanotechnology, said: "The concept of targeted drug delivery is something which has been around for a while and there are many different avenues that have been tested. "This one looks like an interesting and promising one. "I particularly like the fact that these mini-cells, as they call them, seem to be swallowed up by the cancer cells and taken inside the cancer cells, because that is inherently a very powerful way to actually deliver the drug-actually into the cell."

EXPLORING THE CANCER NANOTECHNOLOGY IN CANCER

Nanotechnology offers the unprecedented and paradigm-changing opportunity to study and interact with normal and cancer cells in real time, at the molecular and cellular scales, and during the earliest stages of the cancer process. Through the concerted development of nanoscale devices or devices with nanoscale materials and components, the NCI Alliance for Nanotechnology in Cancer will facilitate in near future their integration within the existing cancer research infrastructure. The Alliance will bring enabling technologies for:

- Imaging agents and diagnostics that will allow clinicians to detect cancer in its earliest stages
- Systems that will provide real-time assessments of therapeutic and surgical efficacy for accelerating clinical translation
- Multifunctional, targeted devices capable of bypassing biological barriers to deliver multiple therapeutic agents directly to cancer cells and those tissues in the microenvironment that play a critical role in the growth and metastasis of cancer
- Agents that can monitor predictive molecular changes and prevent precancerous cells from becoming malignant
- Novel methods to manage the symptoms of cancer that adversely impact quality of life
- Research tools that will enable rapid identification of new targets for clinical development and predict drug resistance

Use of Nanotechnology in Cancer

Nanoscale devices are somewhere from one hundred to ten thousand times smaller than human cells. They are similar in size to large biological molecules ("biomolecules") such as enzymes and receptors. As an example, hemoglobin, the molecule that carries oxygen in red blood cells, is approximately 5 nanometers in diameter. Nanoscale devices smaller than 50 nanometers can easily enter most cells, while those smaller than 20 nanometers can move out of blood vessels as they circulate through the body.

Because of their small size, nanoscale devices can readily interact with biomolecules on both the surface of cells and inside of cells. By gaining access to so many areas of the body, they have the potential to detect disease and deliver treatment in ways unimagined before now. And since biological processes, including events that lead to cancer, occur at the nanoscale at and inside cells, nanotechnology offers a wealth of tools that are providing cancer researchers with new and innovative ways to diagnose and treat cancer.

Nanotechnologies

Work is currently being done to find ways to safely move these new research tools into clinical practice. Today, cancer-related nanotechnology is proceeding on two main fronts: laboratory-based diagnostics and in vivo diagnostics and therapeutics.

Nanotechnology and Diagnostics

Nanodevices can provide rapid and sensitive detection of cancer-related molecules by enabling scientists to detect molecular changes even when they occur only in a small percentage of cells.

Nanotechnology and Cancer Therapy

Nanoscale devices have the potential to radically change cancer therapy for the better and to dramatically increase the number of highly effective therapeutic agents. Nanoscale constructs can serve as customizable, targeted drug delivery vehicles capable of ferrying large doses of chemotherapeutic agents or therapeutic genes into malignant cells while sparing healthy cells, greatly reducing or eliminating the often unpalatable side effects that accompany many current cancer therapies.

Nano Cancer Fix

A new cancer treatment could kill cancer cells without the painful side effects of chemotherapy. Using nanotechnology, scientists may now be able to destroy tumors without killing healthy cells at the same time.

Nanoshells

For people with cancer, chemotherapy, with its painful side effects, is often the worst part of the treatment process. What if there was a noninvasive cancer treatment that could target a tumor and leave the healthy tissue alone? Now, nanotechnology may be on the way to providing just that. Naomi Halas, professor of chemistry and electrical and computer engineering at Rice University created tiny particles called nanoshells, which are 1/1000th the size of a human hair. "If you could see them they would look a lot like malted milk balls, except they are made of different materials," says Halas, "The crunchy core would instead be made of glass and the chocolate coating would instead be made of gold. And that's very important geometry because being able to control the relative size of the two parts of the nanoshell, the core and the shells, allows us to tune the optical properties of that nanoparticle such that we can control what wavelength of light it absorbs, what color of light it absorbs."

Halas reported in the journal Cancer Letters that the nanoshells' ability to capture light and convert it to heat has, in lab tests on mice, destroyed tumors. She and Rice biomedical engineer Jennifer West coat the nanoshells with a substance that binds them to cancer cells, and inject them into tumors. A harmless near-infrared light heats only the nanoshells, which convert the light into heat that destroys tumor cells, without affecting healthy tissue near the tumor.

Halas and West studied 25 mice with tumors that were divided into three groups: one that received no treatment; one that received saline injections and three minutes of exposure to the near-infrared light; and one that received nanoshell injections and a laser applied on the skin above each tumor.

While tumors in the other two groups of mice continued to grow, the tumors in the group that got the nanoshell treatment disappeared within ten days, and those mice remained cancer-free afterwards. "So far we have never seen any adverse reaction to nanoshells in animals," says West. "We've done a lot of testing at this point and all of the results to date look like they're very safe, non-toxic, and bio-compatible."

Halas says nanoshells would have virtually no side effects because they're not interacting with the organism. "They only are active once they're in place at the tumor site and once one shines light through the skin to the actual tumor site and heats that localized region," she says. "So we feel that is something might make a huge difference in terms of the invasiveness-not just the side effects but the overall lack of invasiveness of this sort of treatment. When nanoshells are directly injected into the bloodstream, the body doesn't recognize them. They're coated with specific molecules that essentially make them stealth particles, so they're not recognizable as a foreign object. Also...they're gold and gold is not recognized as a foreign substance by the human body.

If we compare nanoshell-assisted cancer therapy to conventional cancer therapy for example, like chemotherapy, there's a very high likelihood that the type of side effects that people see in conventional therapies would be greatly reduced."

NCI Announcements

The National Cancer Institute (NCI) announced today at a media briefing a new $144.3 million, five-year initiative to develop and apply nanotechnology to cancer. Nanotechnology, the development and engineering of devices so small that they are measured on a molecular scale, has already demonstrated promising results in cancer research and treatment.

"Nanotechnology has the potential to radically increase our options for prevention, diagnosis, and treatment of cancer," said Andrew von Eschenbach, M.D., director of the National Cancer Institute. "NCI's commitment to this cancer initiative comes at a critical time. Nanotechnology supports and expands the scientific advances in genomics and proteomics and builds on our understanding of the molecular underpinnings of cancer. These are the pillars which will support progress in cancer." To carry out this initiative, the NCI, part of the National Institutes of Health, is forming the NCI Alliance for Nanotechnology in Cancer, a comprehensive, integrated initiative encompassing researchers, clinicians, and public and private organizations that have joined forces to develop and translate cancer-related nanotechnology research into clinical practice. "The Alliance lays out a process to safely accelerate the application of nanotechnology to cancer research," said NCI Deputy Director Anna Barker, Ph.D. "Central to this initiative will be multidisciplinary partnerships involving physicists, biologists, clinicians, engineers, and other experts that can translate knowledge on cancer and nanotechnology into clinically useful products." The new NCI Alliance for Nanotechnology in Cancer is one of the first steps in implementing the Cancer Nanotechnology Plan, which was developed over the past 18 months with the input of a broad cross-section of the cancer research and clinical oncology communities. The NCI Alliance consists of four major program activities:

- o Centers of Cancer Nanotechnology Excellence (CCNEs): The primary goal of the CCNEs is to integrate nanotechnology development into basic and applied cancer research. Each center will be affiliated with a NCI Comprehensive Cancer Center, university, or research center of engineering and physical science. By leveraging existing NCI resources, these centers will bridge gaps in the development pipeline from materials discovery to preclinical testing.

- o Multidisciplinary research teams: Given the multidisciplinary nature of nanotechnology research, investigators with basic science and clinical backgrounds will require training to optimize the development and translation of nanotechnologies toward clinical oncology applications. The NCI will initially use existing career development mechanisms to direct talent to this area, create incentives for cross-disciplinary research, and foster collaboration through training.
- o Nanotechnology platforms for cancer research: Over the next five years, investigator-initiated and directed project research will be supported in six key programmatic areas: molecular imaging and early detection, in vivo imaging, reporters of efficacy (e.g., real-time assessment of treatment), multifunctional therapeutics, prevention and control, and research enablers (opening new pathways for research).
- o Nanotechnology Characterization Laboratory (NCL): The NCL will perform and standardize the pre-clinical characterization of nanomaterials developed by researchers from academia, government, and industry. The NCL will serve as a national resource and knowledge base for cancer researchers, and facilitate the accelerated regulatory review and translation of nanomaterials and devices into the clinical realm.

The NCI recently signed a memorandum of understanding and an interagency agreement with the National Institute of Standards and Technology to partner with the NCI in this characterization and standardization effort. The NCI will also be working to expand collaborations with the U.S. Food and Drug Administration (FDA) to help define the critical pathway for nanotechnologies to reach the clinic.

Among the key components of the Cancer Nanotechnology Plan are milestones to measure success over two time periods. Within the first three years, the plan calls for acceleration of projects that hold promise for near-term clinical application. After three years, the Alliance will focus on developing solutions to address more difficult technological and biological problems that have the potential to impact detection and treatment.

"We are already seeing how nanotechnology is transforming our ability to translate research advances into clinical advances," said Samuel Wickline, M.D., Professor of Medicine, Physics and Biomedical Engineering at Washington University, St. Louis, Mo., and NCI grantee for nanotechnology research. "The possibilities are enormous for finding very small cancers far earlier than ever before and treating them with powerful drugs at the tumor site alone, while at the same time reducing any harmful side effects. This initiative will allow us to explore using this technology to its full potential." Recent advances in cancer treatment involving nanotechnology include:

- Liposomes, the "first generation" of nanoscale drug delivery devices, were developed to deliver anticancer therapeutics directly at tumors. Specifically, liposomal doxorubicin is being used to treat certain forms of cancer, while liposomal amphotericin B treats fungal infections often associated with aggressive anticancer treatments.
- Recently, a nanoparticulate formulation of the well-known anticancer compound taxol was submitted to the FDA as a new treatment for advanced-stage breast cancer.

Other clinical applications of nanotechnology have focused on identifying cancer in its earliest stages, visualizing development of the disease, delivering improved therapy to increase the effectiveness and reduce side effects of drugs, and capturing early signals of drug efficacy.

Future of Nanotechnology

Experiments on mice have shown promise for the future of nanotechnology in treating cancer. The research brings doctors one step closer to being able to inject patients with nanoparticles that bore inside tumours and release powerful doses of cancer-killing drugs while leaving the rest of the body unscathed.

After seeing how the mice were cured of human prostate cancer with the technology, cancer specialists gathered at the European Cancer Conference in Paris praised the work as impressive and said they had high hopes for its application to patients.

"There are a lot of candidates for intelligent carriers, and these nanoparticles are among them," said Dr. Gordon McVie, a professor at the European Institute of Oncology in Milan, Italy, who was not involved with the research. Previous designs of nanoparticles have used antibodies to zone in on cancer cells.

"The body's immunodefence system can create antibodies to the therapeutic antibodies, deactivate them and prevent the antibody binding to the right cancer cells. This looks like a step forward," Kerr said. Nanotechnology is the science of manipulating matter smaller than 100 nanometres and taking advantage of properties that are present only at that level, such as conductivity. A nanometre is one-billionth of a metre, or about one-millionth the size of a pin head. The prefix comes from "nanos," the Greek word for dwarf.

Nanotech has been around for several decades, but only now is its potential starting to be realized. Medicine is expected to be one of the fields to benefit most from the technology. In cancer, it is hoped the technology will allow for more precisely targeted drugs and surgery and less toxic chemotherapy.

The study, conducted by scientists at Harvard Medical School and the Massachusetts Institute of Technology, which are pioneering cancer nanotechnology, involved engineering nanoparticles embedded with the cancer drug Taxotere. The particles were then injected directly into human tumours created from prostate cancer cell lines and implanted into the flanks of mice. The mice were watched for 100 days.

The technology being tested involves a nanoparticle made of a hydrogen and carbon polymer with bits of drug bound up in its fabric and attached to a chemical that hones in on cancer cells. The polymer gradually dissolves, exposing the nuggets of drug little by little.

The mice were divided into five groups, including one that had their tumours injected with ineffective saltwater. A second group died after injections of a nanoparticle containing no drugs.

KILLING CANCER CELLS

Nanotechnology has been harnessed to kill cancer cells without harming healthy tissue. The technique works by inserting microscopic synthetic rods called carbon nanotubules into cancer cells. When the rods are exposed to near-infra red light from a laser they heat up, killing the cell, while cells without rods are left unscathed.

Researcher Dr Hongjie Dai said: "One of the longstanding problems in medicine is how to cure cancer without harming normal body tissue."

"Standard chemotherapy destroys cancer cells and normal cells alike. That's why patients often lose their hair and suffer numerous other side effects."

"For us, the Holy Grail would be finding a way to selectively kill cancer cells and not damage healthy ones."

The carbon nanotubules used by the Stanford team are only half the width of a DNA molecule, and thousands can easily fit inside a typical cell. Under normal circumstances near-infra red light passes through the body harmlessly. But the Stanford team found that if they placed a solution of carbon nanotubules under a near-infra red laser beam, the solution heated up to about 70°C in two minutes. They then placed the tubules inside cells, and found they were quickly destroyed by the heat generated by the laser beam.

Dr Dai said: "It's actually quite simple and amazing. We're using an intrinsic property of nanotubes to develop a weapon that kills cancer." The next step was to find a way to introduce the nantubules into cancer cells, but not healthy cells. The researchers did this by taking advantage of the fact that, unlike normal cells, the surface of cancer cells is covered with receptors for a vitamin known as folate. They coated the nanotubules with folate molecules, making it easy for them to pass into cancer cells, but unable to bind with their healthy cousins.

Exposure to the laser duly killed off the diseased cells, but left the healthy ones untouched.

New Advanced Technique

The researchers believe it should be possible to refine the technique still further, for instance by attaching an antibody to a nanotubule to target a particular kind of cancer cell.

Dr Emma Knight, of the charity Cancer Research UK, said: "Nanotechnology has a lot to offer biomedical science, and the results of this paper suggest yet another way in which it may help in the fight against cancer.

"However, this work is still at a very early stage. The researchers have shown that near-infra red light can cause nanotubes to produce heat that can kill cancer cells.

"But their work so far has focused on cells that have been grown in culture in the laboratory.

"Further research will be crucial to see whether these effects can be reproduced in the more complex environment of a tumour and, ultimately, the human body."

CONVERTING CARBON NANOTUBES INTO RNA-DEGRADING NANO-ENZYMES

The researchers and scientists at Rensselaer Polytechnic Institute and the University of Illinois, Urbana-Champaign have achieved a major breakthrough in utilizing nanotechnology. The team of researchers has been successful in combining a DNA-based enzyme with a carbon nanotube; they have successfully combined the DNA based enzyme and have converting Carbon Nanotubes into RNA-Degrading Nano-Enzymes. Thus they have created a nanoscale device capable of degrading specific sequences of RNA.

Such a device is capable of providing a novel approach to treat cancer. This device would be quite a beneficial instrument in cancer therapy as it would be enabling researchers to block a cancer cell's production of proteins needed to maintain a cancerous state.

Carbon nanotubes were at one time the sole province of material scientists and structural engineers. The application of nanotechnology has diversified the use of carbon nanotubes and they have now captured the attention of cancer researchers because of the ability of these nanoscale structures to cross the cell membrane, ferrying in proteins and other potential imaging and drug molecules. A team headed by Jonathan Dordick, Ph.D., is attempting to use this capability to deliver so-called DNAzymes to the cells. DNAzymes are short stretches of single-stranded DNA that break down specific sequences of RNA. The cells use these specific sequences of RNA and thereafter the cells use it to convert information stored in their chromosomes into the myriad proteins they need to thrive.

Numerous experiments have shown that breaking down a specific RNA, and thus turning off production of the corresponding protein, can have a therapeutically beneficial result.

As reported in Journal of the American Chemical Society, the researchers delineate and describe a five-step process for attaching DNAzymes to the surface of a carbon nanotube. The resulting DNAzyme-nanotube hybrid retains all of the enzymatic activity of the DNAzymes without the use of any special reaction conditions, that is, the hybrid would have a good chance of degrading RNA under the conditions found within a cell.

It is quite interesting to note that this hybrid may also be able to simultaneously transport other molecules into cells by packing this secondary payload into the hollow core of the nanotubes. These highly active and stable DNAzyme, which are essentially carbon nanotube hybrids, are major breakthrough into the application of nanotechnology for treatment of cancer.

Custom Nanoparticles Improving Cancer Diagnosis and Treatment

Researchers have developed "custom" nanoparticles that show promise of providing a more targeted and effective delivery of anticancer drugs than conventional medications or any of the earlier attempts to fight cancer with nanoparticles. Designed at the molecular level to attack specific types of cancer without affecting healthy cells, the nanoparticles also have the potential to reduce side effects associated with chemotherapy, the researchers say. Their study was described today at the 231st national meeting of the American Chemical Society, the world?s largest scientific society. The particles, considered the next generation of cancer therapeutics, are the most uniform, shape-specific drug delivery particles developed to date, according to researchers at the University of North Carolina (UNC) in Chapel Hill. Other potential benefits of the tiny uniform particles include enhanced imaging of cancer cells for improved diagnosis and use as delivery vehicles for gene therapy agents, they say.

To date, the UNC researchers have produced a variety of custom nanoparticles from biocompatible organic materials using techniques they adapted from processes used by the electronics industry to make transistors. In cell studies, they have shown that the uniform nanoparticles can attach to specific cell targets, release important chemotherapy drugs inside cells, and hold MRI contrast agents. Animal studies began recently and human studies are anticipated, the researchers say.

"I think this will transform the way one detects and treats disease," says study leader Joseph DeSimone, Ph.D., a chemistry professor at UNC and director of the school's Institute for Advanced Materials, Nanoscience and Technology. He has co-founded a company, Liquidia Technologies, to develop and produce the nanoparticles.

Researchers have been experimenting with nanoparticles as drug delivery vehicles for years but have had only limited success in cell and animal studies, DeSimone says. Each carrier has drawbacks with regard to stability in the bloodstream or ability to be directed toward a specific cancer site. In addition, there has been no general method available that allows precise control of the particle?s size, shape and composition, which are considered key features for the success of targeted drug delivery, he says.

Now, DeSimone and his associates at UNC have developed a new fabrication technique that allows, for the first time, unprecedented control over the structure and function of drug delivery nanoparticles. Called PRINT (Particle Replication In Non-wetting Templates), the technique is similar to injection molding and uses principles borrowed from the electronics industry for transistor fabrication, they say. The technique was first detailed last June in the online version of the Journal of the American Chemical Society.

The manufacturing process starts with a silicon wafer that is etched with the shape and size of the desired nanoparticle, resulting in a template. Next, nonstick liquid fluoropolymers are poured into the template and cured to form a fixed mold. The finished mold is then injected with organic materials that can contain imaging agents, anticancer drugs, DNA (for gene therapy) and other materials, depending on the intended function, DeSimone says. The new manufacturing technique uses gentler processing methods that are less likely to harm important organic components than traditional nanoparticle manufacturing techniques, he adds.

The resulting nanoparticles can be as small as 20 nanometers, or thousands of times smaller than the width of a single human hair. The shapes of the particles can also be made to mimic the shapes of objects found in nature like red blood cells or virus particles, DeSimone says.

NANOTECHNOLOGY-TO TREAT OVARIAN CANCER

Manufacture of stain resistant clothes to light and strong tennis rackets.... The way things are created is being transformed by nanotechnology. But, this technology will have its greatest influence on the healthcare industry in future.

Researchers at Rush University Medical Center in Chicago think that remarkably new ways of diagnosing and treating ovarian cancer can be developed using nanotechnology. Rush researchers are using state-of-the-art nanotechnology to improve women's health. They are working in collaboration with Argonne National Laboratory and the Illinois Institute of Technology.

"While the mortality rates of many cancers have decreased significantly in recent decades, the rate for ovarian cancer had not changed much in the last 50 years, primarily due to delays in diagnosis," said Dr. Jacob Rotmensch, section director of gynecologic oncology at Rush.

"By exploiting the unique properties of nanotechnology, we hope to detect ovarian cancer earlier using highly sensitive imaging tools and develop drug carriers that can deliver therapeutic agents inside tumor cells."

"A nanotechnology based approach is needed because diagnosis of early stage cancer requires the detection and characterization of very small quantities of biomarker," added Dr. Liaohai Chen, a molecular biologist and leader of the nano-bio group in the Biosciences Division at Argonne, and an adjunct faculty at Rush University Medical Center.

A nanometer is one billionth of a meter or 1/80,000 the width of a human hair. Nanoscale devices can perform tasks inside the body that would otherwise not be possible, such as entering most cells and moving through the walls of blood vessels. As a result, nanoscale devices can readily interact with individual molecules on both the cell surface and within the cell, in ways that do not alter the behavior of those molecules.

One area of research involves developing a screening test that would not require removal of the ovary for biopsy. Collaborating with Dr. Rong Wang, an associate professor at Illinois Institute of Technology, the research team is using an atomic force microscope, a very-high resolution microscope that can investigate the interaction of individual protein molecules. With this microscope the research team can study the molecular structure of cancer versus non-cancer cells and compare the stiffness. Cancer tissues are more stiff than healthy tissues. Instead of removing the ovary to determine if cancerous tissue is present, a probe is currently under development to follow the tissue stiffness in vivo to diagnose cancer.

A second area of research involving nanotechnology uses viral particles as templates to fabricate uniform, nanometer imaging probes and drug carriers. The research team is extracting the DNA from viral particles and replacing it with imaging agents.

The goal is to have the viral capsule adhere to a cancer cell and inject the imaging or a therapeutic agent into the cell. This technology could lead to early diagnosis and the development of targeted drug therapy that kills cancer cells while leaving the rest of the body unharmed.

"The development of a smart probe and carrier complex will provide significant advantage to the clinicians as they can locate the tumor, monitor the drug delivery vehicle and control drug release using imaging techniques," said Chen.

Another avenue of nanotechnology research at Rush is to develop nanometer sized contrast agents with ultrasound to diagnose ovarian cancer. Such nano ultrasonographic contrast media can pass through the smallest capillaries. These tiny bubbles light up on ultrasound and may be able to show the earliest vascular changes associated with ovarian malignancy. If this is successful, further research will be conducted to study targeted imaging as well as targeted therapy.

Ovarian cancer is the fifth-most common cancer among American women and claims the lives of more North American women each year than all other gynecologic malignancies combined. About 75 percent of patients are not diagnosed until the disease is in its later stages, and current therapies are not effective enough to successfully treat the disease in such advanced stages.

"There has been a great amount of progress made in the field of nanotechnology over the last five years, but it has not yet been applied to women's health," said Rotmensch. "We believe this 'small-particle' technology has the capability to quickly and sensitively detect cancer molecules earlier than ever before. This research opens new avenues that will directly impact patient care, such as drug development, diagnostic imaging and ultimately, prevention."

NANOTECHNOLOGY IN TREATMENT OF MOUTH CANCER

Nanotechnology is manipulating matter at nanometer level and the application of the same to medicine is called nanomedicine. Nanotechnology holds promise for advanced diagnostics, targeted drug delivery, and biosensors. In the long-term, medical nanorobots will allow instant pathogen diagnosis and extermination, individual cell surgery in vivo, and improvement of natural physiological function.

Current research is focusing on fabrication of nanostructures, nanoactuators, and nanomotors, along with means to assemble them into larger systems, economically and in great numbers.

Science is undergoing yet another change, in helping mankind enter a new era, the era of nanotechnology. "Nano" is derived from the Greek word for 'dwarf. Nanotechnology is the science of manipulating matter measured in the billionths of meters or manometer, roughly the size of 2 or 3 atoms.

In the literature, both a fairly broad as well as a rather narrow concept of nanotechnology are employed. The first signifies any technology smaller than microtechnology. In contrast, the latter stands for the technology to program and manipulate matter with molecular precision and to scale it to 3-D products of arbitrary size.

The basic idea of nanotechnology, used in the narrow sense of the world, is to employ individual atoms and molecules to construct functional structures.

BACKDROP

The late Nobel prize winning physicist Richard P. Feynman in 1959 speculated the potential of nanosize devices as early as 1959. In his historic lecture in 1959, he concluded saying, "this is a development which I think cannot be avoided."

ACHIEVING NANOTECHNOLOGY-PRODUCED GOODS

1. Scientists must be able to manipulate individual atoms.
2. Next step is to develop nanoscopic machines, called assemblers, that can be programmed to manipulate atoms and molecules at will.
3. Inorder to create enough assemblers to build consumer goods, some nanomachines called replicators, will be programmed to build more assemblers.

Assemblers and replicators will work together like hands, to automatically construct products.

PRESENT STATUS

Current research is not exclusively focused on achieving assemblers. Instead, research is directed towards the production of a wide array of different minuscule structures. The fabrication techniques of these structures can be divided into 2 approaches: "top-down" and "bottom--up".

The 'top-down' techniques that are used to manufacture nanoscale structures are mostly extensions of methods already employed in small-scale assembly at the micron scale. By further miniaturization, the nanodimension is entered. 'Bottom-up' fabrication methods for manufacture are the methods used for producing nanoscale structures.

The various nanostructures are:

1. Nanopores
2. Nanotubes
3. Quantumdots
4. Nanoshells
5. Dendrimers

Nanodentistry will make possible the maintenance of near-perfect oral health through the use of nanornaterials, biotechnology including tissue engineering and nanorobotics. Oral health and disease trends may change the focus on specific diagnostic and treatment modalities.

BOTTOM-UP APPROACH

Local Anaesthesia

In the era of nanodentistry a colliodal suspension containing millions of active analgesic micron-size dental robots will be instilled on the patient's gingiva. After contacting the surface of crown or mucosa, the ambulating nanorobots reach the pulp via the gingival sulcus, lamina propria and dentinal tubules. Once installed in the pulp, the analgesic dental robots may be commanded by the dentist to shut down all sensitivity in any particular tooth that requires treatment.

After oral procedures are completed, the dentist orders the nanorobots to restore all sensation, to relinquish control of nerve traffic and to egress from the tooth by similar pathways used for ingress.

Hypersensitivity Cure

Dentin hypersensitivity may be caused by changes in pressure transmitted hydrodynamically to the pulp. This is based on the fact that hypersensitive teeth have 8 times higher surface density of dentinal tubules and tubules with diameters twice as large than nonsensitive teeth. Dental nanorobots could selectively and precisely occlude selected tubules in minutes, using native biological materials, offering patients a quick and permanent cure.

Nanorobotic Dentifrice

Subocclusal dwelling nanorobotic dentifrice delivered by mouthwash or toothpaste could patrol all supragingival and subgingival surfaces atleast once a day, metabolising trapped organic matter into harmless and odorless vapors and performing continuous calculus debridement. These invisibly small dentifrobots [1-10 micon], crawling at 1-10 microns/sec, would be inexpensive, purely mechanical devices, that would safely desactivate themselves if swallowed and would be programmed with strict occlusal avoidance protocol.

Dental Durability and Cosmetics

Tooth durability and appearance may be improved by replacing upper enamel layers with pure sapphire and diamond which can be made more fracture resistant as nanostructured composites, possibly including embedded carbon nanotubes.

Orthodontic Treatment

Orthodontic nanorobots could directly manipulate the periodontal tissues, allowing rapid and painless tooth straightening, rotating and vertical repositioning within minutes to hours.

Photosensitizers and Carriers

Quantum dots can be used as photosensitizers and carriers. They can bind to the antibody present on the surface of the target cell and when stimulated by UV light, they can give rise to reactive oxygen species and thus will be lethal to the target cell.

TOP-DOWN APPROACH

Nanocomposites

Nanoproducts Corporation has successfully manufactured nonagglomerated discrete nanoparticles that are homogeneously distributed in resins or coatings to produce nanocomposites. The nanofiller used includes an aluminosilicate powder having a mean particle size of 80 ran and a 1:4 M ratio of alumina to silica and a refractive index of 1.508.

Advantages

* Superior hardness
* Superior flexural strength, modulus of elasticity and translucency
* 50% reduction in filling shrinkage
* Excellent handling properties

Trade name: Filtek O Supreme Universal Restorative P Lire Nano O

Nanosolution

Nanosolutions produce unique and dispersible nanoparticles, which can be used in bonding agents. This ensures homogeneity and ensures that the adhesive is perfectly mixed everytime.

Trade Name: Adper O Single Bond Plus Adhesive Single Bond

Impression materials

Nanofillers are integrated in vinylpolysiloxanes, producing a unique addition of siloxane impression materials. The material has better flow, improved hydrophilic properties and enhanced detail precision.

Trade Name: Nanotech Elite H-D

Nanoencapsulation

SWRI [South West Research Institute] has developed targeted release systems that encompass nanocapsules including novel vaccines, antibiotics and drug delivery with reduced side effects. At present, targeted delivery of genes and drugs to human liver has been developed by Osaka University in Japan 2003.

Engineered Hepatitis B virus envelope L particles were allowed to form hollow nanoparticles displaying a peptide that is indispensable for liver-specific entry by the virus in humans. Future specialized nanoparticles could be engineered to target oral tissues, including cells derived from the periodontium [Yamada et al, 2003]

Other Products Manufactured by SWRI

a. Protective clothing and filtration masks, using antipathogenic nanoemulsions and nanoparticles
b. Medical appendages for instantaneous healing
    * Biodegradable nanofibres-delivery platform for haemostatic
    * Wound dressings with silk nanofibres in development

* Nanocrystalline silver particles with antimicrobial properties on wound dressings [ActicoatTM, UK]

c. Bone targeting nanocarriers

Calcium phosphate-based biomaterial has been developed. This bone biomaterial is an easily flowable, moldable paste that conforms to and interdigitates with host bone. It supports growth of cartilage and bone cells.

Nanoneedles

Suture needles incorporating nano-sized stainless steel crystals have been developed.

Trade Name: Sandvik Bioline, RK 91TM needles [AB Sandvik, Sweden].

Nanotweezers are also under development which will make cell-surgery possible in the near future.

Bone Replacement Materials

Hydroxyapatite nanoparticles used to treat bone defects are:

* Ostim (Osartis GmbH, Germany) HA
* VITOSSO (Orthovita, Inc, USA) HA +TCP
* NanOSSTM (Angstrom Medica, USA) HA

Nanorobots: Safety Norms

The nonpyrogenicnanorobots used in vivo are bulk teflon, carbon powder and monocrystal sapphire. Pyrogenic nanorobots are alumina, silica and trace elements like copper and zinc. If inherent nanodevice surface pyrogenicity cannot be avoided, the pyrognic pathway is controlled by invivo medical nanorobots.

Nanorobots may release inhibitors, antagonists or dowmegulators for the pyrognic pathway in a targeted fashion to selectively absorb the endogenous pyrogens, chemically modify them, then release them back into the body in a harmless inactivated form.

Challenges for Nanodentistry

* Precise positioning and assembly of molecular scale part
* Economical nanorobot mass production technique
* Biocompatibility
* Simultaneous coordination of activities of large numbers of independent micron-scale robots.
* Social issues of public acceptance, ethics, regulation and human safety

Problems for Research in Nanotechnology in India

* Painfully slow strategic decisions
* Sub-optimal funding
* Lack of engagement ofprivateenterprises
* Problem of retention of trained manpower

FUTURE EXPECTATIONS

Nanotechnology is foreseen to change health care in a fundamental way:

* Novel methods for disease diagnosis and prevention
* Therapeutic selection tailored to the patient's profile
* Drug delivery and gene therapy

2

Advance Light-activated Cancer Nanotech Therapy

Photodynamic therapy (PDT) is a powerful approach for destroying tumors, one that uses light and a light-sensitive chemical to rapidly kill cells. Unfortunately, PDT is associated with significant side effects that largely result from the fact that light-sensitive chemicals, or photosensitizers, distribute themselves throughout the body and thus can damage healthy as well as malignant cells. Another limitation arises because the frequency of light needed to excite the photosensitizers can only pass through a few millimeters of skin.

To reduce or even eliminate PDT's therapy-limiting side effects, researchers are attempting to increase uptake of photosensitizers by tumors and decrease uptake by healthy cells, and to do that investigators are relying heavily on nanoparticles. In a new report, investigators at the State University of New York in Buffalo describe a novel nanoparticle that encapsulates a photosensitizer and a special dye molecule that can absorb light capable of traveling deep into the body and transfer that light energy to the photosensitizer. Tests with cultured cancer cells show that this nanoparticle kills tumor cells.

Paras Prasad, Ph.D., principal investigator of the Multifunctional Nanoparticles in Diagnosis and Therapy of Pancreatic Cancer program, one of National Cancer Institute-funded Cancer Nanotechnology Platform Partnerships, led this research effort. The results of this work appear in the Journal of the American Chemical Society.

The main component of this new system is an organically modified silica nanoparticle that Prasad's group has been developing for several years. Within this nanoparticle, the investigators encapsulated a novel dye molecule that can absorb and emit light in spite of being packed closely to other dye molecules; the optical performance of most dye molecules drops precipitously when they are in close contact with other dye molecules. The nanoparticles also contain a photosensitizer that efficiently absorbs light emitted by this particular dye. This photosensitizer, known as HPPH, recently began to be tested in human clinical trials.

Initial tests with this nanoparticle formulation showed that it generated cell-killing reactive oxygen when irradiated with near-infrared light, the portion of the light spectrum that passes through skin and other tissues easily. Additional experiments showed that tumor cells took in these nanoparticles over a 3-hour period and that when the cells were subsequently irradiated with near-infrared light, the cells died from the internally generated reactive oxygen.

In a second study, published in the journal Molecular Pharmaceutics, the investigators showed that nanocrystals of HPPH could also trigger reactive oxygen production in tumor cells. The purpose of this study was to determine if it was possible to create a formulation of HPPH that is stable in water yet retains its cell-killing activity. HPPH belongs to a category of drugs, which includes many anticancer agents, that are poorly soluble in water. Pure drug nanocrystals dispersed readily in water and were taken up by tumor cells.

TARGETED CANCER THERAPY

Cancer nanotechnology is currently under intense development for applications in cancer imaging, molecular diagnosis and targeted therapy. The basic rationale is that nanometer-sized particles, such as biodegradable micelles, semiconductor quantum dots and iron oxide nanocrystals, have functional or structural properties that are not available from either molecular or macroscopic agents. When linked with biotargeting ligands, such as monoclonal antibodies, peptides or small molecules, these nanoparticles are used to target malignant tumors with high affinity and specificity. In the 'mesoscopic' size range of 5-100 nm in diameter, nanoparticles also have large surface areas and functional groups for conjugating to multiple diagnostic (e.g., optical, radioisotopic or magnetic) and therapeutic (e.g., anticancer) agents. Recent advances have led to multifunctional nanoparticle probes for molecular and cellular imaging, nanoparticle drugs for targeted therapy, and integrated nanodevices for early cancer detection and screening. These developments have opened exciting opportunities for personalized oncology in which cancer detection, diagnosis and therapy are tailored to each individual's molecular profile, and also for predictive oncology, in which genetic/molecular information is used to predict tumor development, progression and clinical outcome.

Cancer Therapy with No side-effects

Most of you know at least one person who has been affected by cancer and treated by chemotherapy, suffering from side-effects such as hair loss or nausea. This is because chemotherapy attacks both healthy and unhealthy cells in the whole body. Now, Australian researchers are using nanotechnology to offer chemotherapy relief. They've created 'nano-cells' from 'inert' bacteria-meaning they can't reproduce-which can deliver potent drugs exactly where they're needed. As this new therapy allows to target very precisely the tumors, the amounts of drugs are much smaller and the harmful side-effects of chemotherapy will be avoided in the future. This method could be used for a wide variety of cancers and human clinical trials should start by the end of this year. Here are some short excerpts of the Agençe France-Presse report.

Researchers there have used bacterial cells stripped of reproductive powers to develop receptacles capable of carrying any chemotherapy drug. These 'nano-cells', which are about one-fifth the size of of normal human cells, are then tagged with antibodies, which are attracted to cancerous tumours. Once the nano-cell hits the cancer and attaches, the drug is released directly into the malignant growth.

As said Jennifer MacDiarmid of Sydney-based biotechnology company EnGeneIC, "Your hair wouldn't fall out, you wouldn't throw up... some chemotherapy is life-threatening in itself." And she added that with their new method, "There is no other system where you can get so much drug concentrated into a little parcel."

In "Cancer therapy cuts side effects," BBC News adds more details about the future of this method.

It is hoped the technique could treat tumours in the breast, ovaries, colon and lungs. So far it has been used in mice and dogs, and the researchers plan to begin human trials shortly. In tests, the technique reduced tumours in animals without side effects-and by using only a very small amount of drug. Dr MacDiarmid said the treatment could potentially be used on any solid tumours.

In "'Mini-cells' could stop side-effects of chemotherapy," New Scientist asks the question: "Could bacteria be the future of cancer therapy?" And it describes what the researchers have done with bacteria.

When bacteria divide, they normally do so at their centres. But Himanshu Brahmbhatt and Jennifer MacDiarmid, of EnGeneIC in Sydney, Australia, have found a way of forcing them to divide at their ends, producing small buds of cytoplasm each time. They have also discovered that a range of different drugs could be packaged into these particles. These "mini bacteria", or EnGeneIC Delivery Vehicles (EDVs) as the company has dubbed them, are cheap and easy to produce, and can be used as targeted drug delivery vehicles.

"They look like bacteria but they have no chromosomes and are non-living," says MacDiarmid. "And because they have a rigid membrane they don't break down when injected, so they carry their payload happily to the target site."

Systemic administration of chemotherapeutic agents results in indiscriminate drug distribution and severe toxicity. Here we report a technology potentially overcoming these shortcomings through encapsulation and cancer cell-specific targeting of chemotherapeutics in bacterially derived 400 nm minicells. We discovered that minicells can be packaged with therapeutically significant concentrations of chemotherapeutics of differing charge, hydrophobicity, and solubility.

These findings have also recently been presented by Himanshu Brahmbhatt, Joint CEO, EnGeneIC Pty Ltd, at the RNAi 2007 conference held in Boston, Massachusetts, on May 3, 2007. By scrolling down through this page, you'll discover the abstract of the presentation named "Turning siRNA into a cancer therapeutic: Bacterially-derived non-living nanoparticles for the targeted delivery of siRNA and shRNA for potent anti-tumor effects in vivo." [Note: siRNA is a shortcut for Small interfering RNA, as described by Wikipedia.] Below is a comment about how these nanoparticles, dubbed as EDVs (EnGeneIC Delivery Vehicles), are acting.

We discovered that EDVs can be packaged with therapeutically significant concentrations of siRNAs as well as chemotherapeutic drugs of differing charge, hydrophobicity and solubility. Targeting of EDVs via bispecific antibodies (BsAbs) to receptors on cancer cell membranes results in endocytosis, intracellular degradation and release of the payload. Intact and fully functional siRNAs are released intracellularly to achieve target mRNA knockdown resulting in highly significant anti-tumor effects as well as drug resistance reversal.

3-D Model of Breast Cancer

The reaserchers of U.K. have built a 3-D version of breast cancer in a test tube. Their model contains cells from normal and cancerous breast tissue. The researchers used a collagen gel to form 3-D structures to create structures similar to the ones find in a woman breast. So far, they focused on a common pre-cancerous condition known as 'ductal carcinoma in situ' (DCIS). With this model, they hope to reduce experiments done on animals such as mice. In fact, these experiments are not always useful because similarities can be poor between mice and humans. Now it remains to be seen if this model will be endorsed by the scientific community.

Before going further, here is a definition of what is DCIS: "Ductal carcinoma in situ (DCIS) is a condition that can occur in several different forms. In all of these, there is a change in the cells lining the milk ducts of the breast. Under a microscope, a normal duct shows a lining of a single layer of cells, but in DCIS, many more cells can be seen. [...] These extra cells in the duct show some of the abnormalities of cancer cells, but they have not spread outside the duct (in situ means 'in place'). For this reason, DCIS is not considered to be 'true' or invasive cancer." Below is a diagram of a breast cross section showing ducts without and with DCIS (Credit for image and caption: The Cancer Council Victoria, Australia)

This project has been led by Louise Jones, professor of breast pathology at the Institute of Cancer at Queen Mary, University of London. Here are some of our explanations about this project.

Jones said "that they needed to develop a test tube model that was more complex than a layer of cells in a Petri dish. Instead the team grew three types of cells from normal and cancerous breast tissue. And using a collagen gel to form three-dimensional structures they have been able to create structures which closely resemble the ways the cells would be organised in the breast."

But how this 3-D Model Help in Cancer Research?

Professor Jones said working out why the cells behave like this could help doctors decide which patients with early cancer to treat and pave the way for developing new treatments. The model could also replace the need for some experiments which are done in animals such as mice, which can be implanted with human tumours.

This is where my interest was growing. Is this research done for the interest of women or mice? In fact, this research is being funded by the Dr Hadwen Trust for an amount of £105,000. And "the Dr Hadwen Trust is the UK's leading medical research charity that funds and promotes exclusively non-animal research techniques to replace animal experiments." So let's look at the press release they issued on May 10, 2007, "Breast cancer in a test tube could replace animal tests."

Breast cancer research is often conducted in mice, with up to 400 mice used in a series of tests. Each animal is likely to endure up to eight separate tumour implants followed by painful drug injections into the abdomen, and distressing, serial 'harvesting' of subsequent tumours. As well as causing suffering, these mouse experiments are potentially misleading, meaning a human-based research approach is vital to improve accuracy.

As says Nicky Gordon, Science Officer for the Dr Hadwen Trust: "As a medical research charity we aim to alleviate human suffering, but we believe that medical excellence can and should be achieved without causing animals suffering too. With breast cancer, there is an urgent need to move away from animal research models because their similarity to human cancer can be so poor.

NEW TOOLS IN NANOTECHNOLOGY

The medical school's close partnership with Georgia Tech, together with grants from the NIH and Georgia Research Alliance, is enabling advances in the study of biologic systems on the molecular level. A $19 million grant from the National Cancer Institute to Emory and Georgia Tech created a National Center of Cancer Nanotechnology Excellence (CCNE), one of seven in the country. The CCNE serves as a "discovery accelerator" to integrate nanotechnology into early detection as well as personalized treatments of cancer. This grant builds on earlier NIH funding (almost $10 million) to develop nanoparticle quantum dot probes to detect biomarkers for early cancer and to monitor the effects of cancer therapy.

Emory and Georgia Tech also received an earlier NIH grant of $11.5 million to use nanotechnology to analyze cardiovascular plaque formation at the molecular level and to detect it at its earliest stages.

Most recently, the NIH and the Georgia Research Alliance awarded shared grants that could total as much as $10 million over five years to Georgia Tech, Emory, and the Medical College of Georgia to create a center to study DNA repair.

VACCINE DEVELOPMENT AND STRATEGIES

Vaccines against HIV-One of the largest and most successful academic vaccine centers in the world, the Emory Vaccine Center, based at the Yerkes National Primate Research Center, was the first U.S. university-based center to have an HIV/AIDS vaccine candidate in human clinical trials. This vaccine, which uses bits of DNA from HIV to prime the immune response, followed by a boost from poxvirus also carrying HIV DNA, recently entered a new trial at sites around the country to evaluate safety and immune responses at low and high doses and to determine optimal dosing schedules. The vaccine center also recently received a $4.5 million grant for its work in vaccine adjuvants from the Bill & Melinda Gates Foundation's Collaboration for AIDS Vaccine Discovery.

The vaccine center is also partnering with an agency founded by the World Health Organization in New Delhi, India, the International Center for Genetic Engineering and Biotechnology, to develop and help move vaccines from the laboratory through the complex testing, approval, and manufacturing process to local health centers in Indian towns and villages hard hit by HIV.

Vaccines against hepatitis C-A $12.5 million grant from the Grand Challenges in Global Health Initiative, also funded by the Gates Foundation, recognizes the promise of a new immunologic blockade strategy developed at the Emory Vaccine Center to reduce the staggering health and economic impact of hepatitis C. The most common bloodborne viral disease in the United States, hepatitis C affects 170 million people worldwide, with little treatment available in the developing world.

Working with the immune-suppressed-A longstanding collaboration between the directors of the Emory Transplant Center and the Emory Vaccine Center is so productive that the NIH sometimes calls for relationship advice to pass on to other less amicably functioning research teams. This year, the National Institute of Allergy and Infectious Diseases awarded $10 million to the team, in collaboration with the Yerkes National Primate Research Center, to develop new vaccine strategies that can better protect organ transplant recipients and other immune-suppressed patients from threats of infectious disease.

The NIH wants to know how to protect these severely immunosuppressed patients-and the rapidly expanding groups of patients with immune systems partially suppressed by chronic viral or autoimmune diseases or by chemotherapy-from the triple threats of bioterrorism, emerging infectious diseases, and the ever-present possibility of a new influenza pandemic. Immunosuppressed people also represent a sizeable hole in any national and global containment strategies against bioterrorism or emerging infectious disease.

New Directions in Transplantation

Emory's Juvenile Diabetes Research Foundation (JDRF) Center recently received new funding of almost $8.5 million from the JDRF to continue work on advancing islet transplant to restore insulin production as a mainstream therapy for type 1 diabetes. The new funding applies to several projects, including testing of a new immunosuppressant drug in human trials and use of xenotransplantation, or islets transplanted from other species, in nonhuman primates.

Emory's transplant team is a world leader in developing and testing improved immunosuppressant drugs, first in primates at Yerkes and then in humans, to help patients better tolerate transplanted organs or tissue. These drugs block the body's immune response more selectively than traditional immunosuppressive drugs and with less toxicity.

The Drug Development

When the NIH decided to fund a national network of molecular screening centers, able to screen hundreds of thousands of compounds against protein targets using high-throughput robotics equipment, Emory was already up and running with its own screening lab. An Emory University Chemical-Biology Discovery Center, made up of faculty from the departments of pharmacology and chemistry and from the Winship Cancer Institute, placed Emory squarely on the front line of academic drug screening. Emory's history in successful AIDS drug discovery and a track record of collaboration between the medical school and the university's chemistry department also gave Emory a leg up in the selection process for the new NIH screening center.

Last year, Emory was designated one of nine new centers in the NIH Molecular Libraries Screening Center Network, with a grant of $9 million, including a library of 100,000 molecular compounds, almost doubling the number already available at Emory.

One protein now under study at Emory enables cell-to-cell communication that triggers cancer oncogenes. Another interacts with the BRCA1 protein involved in breast cancer. Finding compounds to inhibit these proteins could prevent or slow the growth of tumors.

Fragile X: Prevalence and New Drugs

Geneticist Stephen Warren has built the world's most extensive research program on fragile X syndrome, the leading cause of inherited mental retardation. Now the search is on for a drug treatment.

Recent work by the Emory team pointed to what would be needed in a drug to reactivate production of the protein that is missing in fragile X. Warren and his colleagues then identified compounds that work in fruit flies and mice. In an effort to fast-track drugs that can help human patients, they now are screening every drug ever approved by the FDA, more than 2000, looking for one or more with the same capabilities of these other compounds. They have identified several already and are confident that, with the safety and efficacy studies already completed for these drugs, clinical trials for fragile X patients can proceed rapidly.

Under a grant from the Centers for Disease Control and Prevention, other team members are using a novel technology developed at Emory to determine the true incidence of fragile X by screening samples from approximately 70,000 newborns in Georgia, using the dried blood samples left over from Georgia's Newborn Screening Program, which currently screens for more than 50 inherited metabolic disorders. The team hopes that fragile X can become part of routine newborn screening, allowing early intervention and support and eventually, use of new therapies under development.

Alzheimer's Disease: Earlier Diagnosis and Treatment

Recently designated an Alzheimer's Disease Research Center by the National Institute of Aging, Emory joins an elite network of 32 centers nationwide. The designation was accompanied by a $7.4 million grant to the schools of medicine, nursing, and public health and to the Yerkes National Primate Research Center, all players in Emory's broad clinical and research programs in Alzheimer's. These programs focus on diagnosing the disease as early as possible and halting its progress. Researchers have already developed new diagnostic tools, including a pharmaceutical compound discovered at Emory and used in conjunction with 3-D PET scans to visualize beta amyloid plaques in a living person. The compound is the first shown to be clinically useful. With a half-life of eight hours, the compound could be distributed widely to clinics and hospitals. The only other such agent known to work has a half-life of 20 minutes, making it impractical for use outside the lab.

A New way of Looking at the Human Genome

In research funded by the National Human Genome Research Institute, Emory scientists recently identified and created a map of more than 400,000 insertions and deletions (INDELs) in the human genome. INDELs are a little-explored type of genetic variation among individuals, different from the much-studied single nucleotide polymorphisms or SNPs.

INDELs result from the insertion and deletion of small pieces of DNA of varying sizes and types. If SNPs (single chemical bases in the genome sequence) are analogous to single letter changes in the genome "instruction book," then INDELs are equivalent to insertion and deletion of whole words or paragraphs. Both SNPs and INDELs are likely to have a major impact on health and susceptibility to disease. At present, biochemist Scott Devine and his colleagues expect to expand their map of 400,000 INDELs to between 1 and 2 million in the near future.

Emory's partnerships with institutions like the CDC and Georgia Tech leverage research investments to yield faster and bigger payoff.

Increasing the Success of Lung Cancer Therapy

The National Cancer Institute recently awarded $7.9 million to the Winship Cancer Institute to support 40 researchers and clinicians from 10 departments throughout the medical school and university who are involved in multiple studies seeking new drugs that interfere with signaling between cancer cells. Under the NCI grant, which is one of the largest lung cancer research grants in the country, the researchers hope to exploit the abnormalities of lung cancer signaling and identify novel compounds that target an oncogene to battle the proliferation of lung cancer cells. Similar approaches have proven successful for leukemia and HER2-type breast cancer. The researchers also seek to better predict which patients will benefit from chemotherapy and thus help clinicians make more informed clinical decisions, another step toward individualizing therapy for cancer patients.

Fighting Health Disparities

Triple-negative breast cancers-ones that respond to blockage of none of the three more well-known substances that can cause breast tumors to grow (estrogen, progesterone, and HER-2/neu)-tend to strike younger women and occur twice as frequently in African American women as in others. Emory researcher Mary Jo Lund was part of the multi-institutional team that reported the racial difference in incidence this past year. She is working now to establish a repository of tumor specimens from all women newly diagnosed with breast cancer in Fulton and DeKalb counties, where 20% of all breast cancers in Georgia are diagnosed. Black female residents of these counties account for 38% of all newly diagnosed invasive breast cancers, and an inordinately large proportion of these women are under 50 when diagnosed. Lund hopes to use the data she gathers to improve outcomes for all women with breast cancer, particularly the underserved. The medical school also focuses on health disparities in other diseases. The National Heart, Lung and Blood Institute recently awarded $6 million to Emory's medical and nursing schools, working in conjunction with Morehouse School of Medicine, to address health disparities in people at risk for developing cardiovascular disease.

CANCER NANOTECH

Think small-really small. Nanotechnology employs devices with dimensions of one to 1,000 nanometers. To put this in perspective, consider the following: a nanometer is 1/80,000th the width of a human hair; it is the length of 10 hydrogen atoms placed end to end; and it is less than one third the height of a single twist on a strand of DNA. At these sizes it is no wonder that scientists have seized upon nanotechnology for myriad medical applications.

After all, the human body is built upon a foundation of nature-made nanostructures-genes, proteins, cells-that may be best approached on their own scale. Cancer is the key area of medical nanotechnology research. In the not too distant future, dozens of intriguing nanodevices such as the nanotubes at left may transform cancer diagnosis, treatment, and prevention.-Lexi Krock

Nanotubes

Nanotubes are hollow cylinders made of carbon atoms. Doctors could someday use them as miniscule syringes for injecting cells with drugs from within the body, or as nanoscale diagnostic probes the patient would never feel. They can also be filled and sealed, forming test tubes or potential drug delivery devices.

Here, an array of nanotubes engage in what their creators at the Oak Ridge National Laboratory call "impalefection," the capturing of genetic materials by impaling cells (a hamster's ovary cells in this case). In the future, nanotubes could help identify DNA mutations associated with a risk of cancer.

Nanowire

This glowing silica nanowire is wrapped around a single strand of human hair. It looks delicate-it is about five times smaller than a virus-but it is several times stronger than spider silk. Researchers have developed coated nanowires that bind to certain proteins that can indicate the presence of prostate cancer before conventional tests can. Other potential applications for nanowires include the early sensing of breast and ovarian malignancies. Nanowires are so small that doctors could one day implant them into the body as permanent health detectives that continuously monitor molecular levels.

Nanocantilever

The honeycomb mesh behind this tiny carbon cantilever is the surface of a fly's eye. Cantilevers are beams anchored at only one end. In the nanoworld, they function as sensors ideal for detecting the presence of extremely small molecules in biological fluids.

Arrays of nanocantilevers coated with antibodies, for example, will bend from the changes in surface tension when substrates that signal a malignancy bind to it. Simply by monitoring whether or not such nanocantilevers are bent, specialists may someday be able to identify the presence of cancer molecules that today are difficult to detect.

Nanoshells

Nanoshells are hollow silica spheres covered with gold. Scientists can attach antibodies to their surfaces, enabling the shells to target certain cells such as cancer cells. In mouse tests, Naomi Halas's research team at Rice University directed infrared radiation through tissue and onto the shells, causing the gold to superheat and destroy tumor cells while leaving healthy ones intact.

Technicians can control the amount of heat with the thickness of the gold and the kind of laser. Nanoshells could one day also be filled with drug-containing polymers. Heating them would cause the polymers to release a controlled amount of the drug. Human trials using gold nanoshells are slated to begin in a couple of years.

Quantum Dots

Quantum dots are miniscule semiconductor particles that can serve as signposts of certain types of cells or molecules in the body. They can do this because they emit different wavelengths of radiation depending on the type of cadmium used in their cores: cadmium sulfide for ultraviolet to blue, cadmium selenide (seen here) for most of the visible spectrum, and cadmium telluride for the far red and near-infrared. (A dot's size determines its precise color within each range.) A polymer coating enables researchers to attach molecules such as antibodies that will seek out and attach to tumors and other targeted cells. The coating also shields nearby cells from the cadmium's toxicity. The different colors of quantum dots provide a powerful tool for labeling and monitoring multiple cells and molecules simultaneously.

NANOPORES

Nanopores have cancer research and treatment applications. Engineered into particles, they are holes that are so tiny that DNA molecules can pass through them one strand at a time, allowing for highly precise and efficient

DNA sequencing. As a DNA strand moves through a nanopore, scientists can monitor each "letter" on it, deciphering coded information, including mutations associated with cancer. By engineering nanopores into the surface of a drug capsule that are only slightly larger than the medicine's molecular structure, drug manufacturers can also use nanopores to control the rate of a drug's diffusion in the body.

THE GOLD NANOPARTICLES

These nanoparticles, seen in a transmission electron micrograph image, are similar in structure to nanoshells, but they have a solid core. Researchers at Northwestern University are using gold nanoparticles to develop ultrasensitive detection systems for DNA and protein markers associated with many forms of cancer, including breast and prostate cancer. The scientists can release swarms of nanoparticles linked to a host of cancer-related antibodies. The nanoparticles can hunt for hundreds of different cancer targets simultaneously. Their tests with cancer molecules in solution revealed that gold nanoparticles are up to one million times as sensitive as conventional cancer-detection approaches.

LIPOSOMES

Liposomes-tiny pouches made of lipids, or fat molecules, surrounding a water core-were the first type of nanoparticles widely used for clinical cancer treatment. Several different kinds of liposomes are also widely employed against infectious diseases and can deliver certain vaccines. During cancer treatment they encapsulate drugs, shielding healthy cells from their toxicity, and prevent their concentration in vulnerable tissues such as those of a patient's kidneys and liver. Liposomes can also reduce or eliminate certain common side effects of cancer treatment such as nausea and hair loss.

Fullerenes

These crystalline particles are a form of carbon atom whose molecular architecture is arranged in a soccer ball-like structure. Also known as buckyballs, they were discovered in 1985 among the detritus of laser-vaporized graphite. Unlike other molecules that have applications as cancer drug delivery vehicles, fullerenes don't break down in the body and are excreted intact. This trait can be important for some cancer treatment compounds that are dangerous to healthy cells. For example, fullerene drug delivery particles that contain radioactive atoms would allow for the complete removal of radiation from the body following treatment.

Dendrimer

This fascinating particle holds significant promise for cancer treatment. Its many branches allow other molecules to easily attach to its surface. Researchers at the University of Michigan have fashioned dendrimers into sophisticated anti-cancer machines carrying five chemical tools-a molecule designed to bind to cancer cells, a second that fluoresces upon locating genetic mutations, a third to assist in imaging tumor shape using X-rays, a fourth carrying drugs released on demand, and a fifth that would send a signal when cancerous cells are finally dead. The creators of these dendrimers have had successful tests with cancer cells in culture and plan to try them in living animals soon.

HUMAN HEALTH AND MEDICINE

NIH is supporting the development of effective, high output, informative, and less costly systems and has identified several areas for research in nanomedicine, which it defines as integration of nanotechnology and medicine. NIH is planning to support the research on biological molecules such as proteins, DNA, and RNA as well as research into how these molecules interact with each other and with environmental agents. One of its primary objectives is acquisition of a comprehensive database and development of quantitative nanomaterial measurements, said Olden. NIH researchers and independent scientists have identified the need for mathematical and analytical tools to quantify manipulations and interpret measurements of nanomolecules. Thus, mathematicians and chemists need to get involved in the effort to understand what these variations, changes, and readouts mean to biological processes.

> *Once an early biomarker of a disease or dysfunction is identified, then scientists can use targeted pharmaceutical or gene therapy to correct the faulty components. — Kenneth Olden*

Additionally, NIH is planning to develop very sensitive detection systems that would be able to detect a single cell or a few cells that are diseased or perturbation of a pathway. Once an early biomarker of a disease or dysfunction is identified, then scientists can use targeted pharmaceutical or gene therapy to correct the faulty components, noted Olden.

Pebble Chemistry as an Example of a Medical Application of Nanotechnology

Nanotechnology, especially as it is applied to biological systems, is an intricate, interdisciplinary field, said Martin Philbert of the University of

Michigan. Researchers have begun to build nanoparticles that are intrinsically biocompatible, that do not alert the immune system to their presence, and that can contain a variety of highly functional and highly specific elements that might be toxic but which are shielded from the biology by a shell. One example, the Probes Encapsulated by Biologically Localized Embedding (PEBBLE) was created as a nanoparticle platform with multi-functional capabilities.

Generally, PEBBLEs are fluorescent dyes that are encased in a molecular shell, protecting cells from the dye and protecting the dye from cellular degradation or manipulation, stated Philbert. The presence and intensity of the fluorescence is directly proportional to the pathway or molecule that the sensor is measuring. Currently, they are being used in research facilities and offer researchers the ability to measure real-time binding, translocation, and molecule production, instead of the widely used tools available for steady-state or endpoint measurements. However, they may have use for a wide range of research and medical needs.

PEBBLE Chemistry

The simplest iteration of a PEBBLE is a polymer shell that contains a fluorescent molecule, ranging in size from 20 nanometers to 600 nanometers in diameter. One 20 nanometer particle occupies 1 thousandth of a human motor neuron in the anterior horn of the spinal cord; thus, cells have a potentially tremendous capacity for the retention of a wide range of PEBBLEs sensing and reporting on a variety of cellular pathways and processes.

Philbert stated that the analytical chemistry that can be performed within the conserved space of the cell is much more sophisticated. A dye can be incorporated that changes with time as a function of the analyte of interest. The system can also be constructed in a more complex fashion using ionophores. When irradiated with the appropriate wavelength of a laser, light is emitted and can be measured, allowing for an amazingly useful property where the measurement system is completely calibratable and the fluorescence is reversible, said Philbert.

PEBBLES as Stepping Stones to Understanding Cellular Processes

One aspect of nanoparticle research has focused on the use of nanoparticles as sensors of cellular activity. This can include extra cellular measurements, such as the presence of oxygen or nitrogen radicals in the extra cellular space and the presence of the molecules in the blood and tissue, or measurements at the subcellular level. Protein movement, oxidation or reduction reactions, and the production of super oxide ions within the cell may be tracked by the use of fluorescent nanoparticles. There are also design prototypes for measuring lead and mercury, and soon, according to Philbert, the ability to measure phosphorylation and other chemical reactions inside the cell will be possible.

The light emitted from individual nanoprobes introduced into the volume of the cell can be viewed using confocal microscopy. The concentration of oxygen at each individual point is reported by a dot in the co-focal viewing field when observing the cell. The intensity of the light emitted by the dot indicates the concentration of oxygen at that point in the cell. With this new look at the cell, Philbert suggested that our assumptions about how oxygen enters the cell, diffuses through the cell, and is used in the cell may not be entirely correct.

Nanoparticles can also be used to track the movement of particular cellular compartments. Endosomes can take up the nanoparticle, and depending on surface charge, size, and other characteristics, transport them to the apical surface or the basal lateral surface of the cell.

The reason why scientists have attempted to go smaller and smaller is that they were trying to find out if there is a point at which the sensors that are being designed and placed into systems to measure biological activity begin affecting or changing the very processes they are intended to measure. Once a molecule is below 100 nanometers, it begins interacting with proteins, potentially signaling proteins, and can result in entirely unintended consequences, which is why PEBBLEs have been kept close to 100, and less than 200, nanometers. Thus while there are many advantages to keeping PEBBLES very small, scientists really do not know yet what the interactions with proteins and other elements of the cell are going to be, said Philbert.

With this new look at the cell our assumptions about how oxygen enters the cell, diffuses through the cell, and is used in the cell may not be entirely correct. — *Martin Philbert*

PEBBLEs on the Path to Understanding Tumor Biology

One area of research, according to Philbert, focuses on targeting molecules to tumors for treatment and eradication. Coating a PEBBLE nanoparticle with a magnetically responsive metal allows researchers to target nanoparticles to specific locations within the body and to obtain a better image of tumors from magnetic resonance imaging (MRI). These MRI images reveal a significant contrast enhancement due to the presence of the nanoparticles within the tumor tissue, that is, nanoparticles allow for very good contrast from normal tissue, where the tumor becomes clearly visible to the observer.

Fine resolution of small tumors is not the only possibility within the same nanoparticle. Ruthenium (Sol Gel Ru-DNPs) can also be included within the nanoparticle. When a laser is turned on, Sol Gel Ru-DNPs can produce a large amount of singlet oxygen only when it reaches the target, in this case a brain tumor called 9L gliosarcoma produced in the rat brain. Therefore, researchers can kill this clone of the gliosarcoma, which does not respond to chemotherapy or radiation therapy. Coupled with a fiber optic that is only a millimeter in diameter, the tumor can be stopped or at least reduced in size with time. Because the 9L gliosarcoma is extremely aggressive, if one or two cells are left, after some time the tumor will re-grow. However, with a single injection and only 10 minutes of laser irradia-

> *The ultimate goal of this research is to create particles that are not going to interfere with the normal biology of the organism and are going to have very high therapeutic index. -Martin Philbert*

Nanoparticles used in tumor killing experiments are larger than 100 nanometers; thus, they do not cross the blood-brain barrier (BBB), and therefore are excluded from healthy brain tissue, said Philbert. These nanoparticles penetrate into the tumor only when a tumor changes the porosity of the blood vessel. This process of BBB penetration takes approximately 5-10 minutes and once clearance through renal and other mechanisms is considered to be complete, the laser is turned on. The nanoparticles are delivered systemically and then pass through the BBB before a laser is turned on to activate the killing activity, but further research will be need to understand what happens to these particles as they circulate through other parts of the body? Approximately twenty different kinds of these nanoparticles have been created and researched in vivo in the Philbert lab alone, all of which have shown effects on the reticular endothelial system and the kidneys. These nanoparticles are discarded as the ultimate goal of this research is to create particles that are not going to interfere with the normal biology of the organism, yet have a very high therapeutic index. Philbert suggested that many of the products that can be created will ultimately not be deployable because early safety testing will show them to be completely unfeasible from a toxicological standpoint.

CANCER TREATMENT WITHOUT HARMING HEALTHY TISSUE

Scientists at Stanford University have developed a new laser therapy that destroys cancer cells but leaves healthy ones unharmed. The new, non-invasive treatment is described in a study published in the Aug. 1 online edition of the Proceedings of the National Academy of Sciences (PNAS).

"One of the longstanding problems in medicine is how to cure cancer without harming normal body tissue," says Hongjie Dai, an associate professor of chemistry at Stanford and co-author of the study. "Standard chemotherapy destroys cancer cells and normal cells alike. That's why patients often lose their hair and suffer numerous other side effects. For us, the Holy Grail would be finding a way to selectively kill cancer cells and not damage healthy ones."

For the PNAS experiment, Dai and his colleagues used a basic tool of nanotechnology-carbon nanotubes, synthetic rods that are only half the width of a DNA molecule. Thousands of nanotubes could easily fit inside a typical cell.

"An interesting property of carbon nanotubes is that they absorb near-infrared light waves, which are slightly longer than visible rays of light and pass harmlessly through our cells," Dai says. But shine a beam of near-infrared light on a carbon nanotube, and the results are dramatic. Electrons in the nanotube become excited and begin releasing excess energy in the form of heat.

In the experiment, Stanford researchers found that if they placed a solution of carbon nanotubes under a near-infrared laser beam, the solution would heat up to about 158 degrees F (70 C) in two minutes. When nanotubes were placed inside cells and radiated by the laser beam, the cells were quickly destroyed by the heat. However, cells without nanotubes showed no effects when placed under near-infrared light.

"It's actually quite simple and amazing," Dai observes. "We're using an intrinsic property of nanotubes to develop a weapon that kills cancer."

Trojan Horse

To assure that only diseased cells were destroyed in the experiment, the scientists had to find a way to selectively deliver carbon nanotubes into cancer cells and not into healthy ones. Dai and his co-workers achieved this by performing a bit of biochemical trickery. Unlike normal cells, the surface of a cancer cell contains numerous receptors for a vitamin known as folate. The researchers decided to coat the nanotubes with folate molecules, which would only be attracted to diseased cells with folate receptors.

The experiment worked as predicted. Most of the folate-coated nanotubes ended up inside cancer cells, bypassing the normal cells-like Trojan horses crossing the enemy line. Once the nanotubes were planted inside, the researchers shined the near-infrared laser on the cancer cells, which soon heated up and died. "Folate is just an experimental model that we used," Dai says. "In reality, there are more interesting ways we can do this. For example, we can attach an antibody to a carbon nanotube to target a particular kind of cancer cell."

One example is lymphoma, or cancer of the lymphatic system. Like many cancers, lymphoma cells have well-defined surface receptors that recognize unique antibodies.

When attached to a carbon nanotube, the antibody would play the role of a Trojan horse. Dai and Dean Felsher, a lymphoma researcher in the Stanford School of Medicine, have begun a collaboration using laboratory mice with lymphoma. The researchers want to determine if shining near-infrared light on the animal's skin will destroy lymphatic tumors, while leaving normal cells intact.

"It's a really interesting idea," says Felsher, an assistant professor of medicine and of pathology. "For a long time people have thought about ways to target cancer cells, and this is a very promising technique."

Researchers at Rice University recently conducted a similar experiment on mice with cancerous tumors. Instead of carbon nanotubes, the Rice team injected the tumors with gold-coated nanoshells and exposed the animals to near-infrared light for several minutes. The tumors disappeared within 10 days without damaging any healthy tissue.

Future Applications

Dai points out that the carbon nanotubes also can be delivered to diseased cells by direct injection.

"In breast cancer, for example, there might come a time when we inject nanotubes into the tumor and expose the breast to near-infrared light," he says. This benign therapy could potentially eliminate months of debilitating chemotherapy and radiation treatment, he adds.

"The laser we used is a 3-centimeter beam that's held like a flashlight," he notes. "We can take the beam and put anywhere we want. We can shine it on a local area of the skin or inside an internal organ using a fiber-optic device."

Dai has applied for a patent on the procedure through Stanford's Office of Technology Licensing (OTL). He also has patented another technique that's designed to deliver molecules of DNA, RNA or protein directly into the cell nucleus to fight various infections and diseases. That method uses pulses of near-infrared light to shake the therapeutic molecule loose from the nanotube after they have entered the cell.

"Nanotechnology has long been known for its applications in electronics," Dai concludes. "But this experiment is a wonderful example of nanobiotechnology-using the unique properties of nanomaterials to advance biology and medicine."

Dai's graduate student, Nadine Wong Shi Kam, is lead author of the PNAS study. Other co-authors are Michael O'Connell, a former postdoctoral fellow in the Department of Chemistry, and graduate student Jeffrey A. Wisdom in the Department of Applied Physics.

The study was partly supported by the National Science Foundation Center on Polymer Interfaces and Macromolecular Assemblies, a research partnership among Stanford, IBM Almaden Research Center, University of California-Davis and University of California-Berkeley.

NON-INVASIVE METHODS

Over the past three decades since the beginning of the National Cancer Initiative in 1971, there have been major advances in the diagnosis and treatment of cancer. However, the ravages of cancer continue to be a major healthcare concern of our society and nation.

As Dr. Eschenbach, Director of the National Cancer Institute stated in September 2004, "... in spite of those opportunities and those breakthroughs, the painful reality is that as we sit here today, one American every minute continues to die from this disease. It remains the disease that Americans fear most because of the suffering and devastation as well as death it brings, and we know that one out of every two men, and one out of every three women in their lifetime will be told they have cancer."

Current treatments by radiation and chemotherapy are also extremely invasive with excruciating side effects. Nanotechnology promises new methods for noninvasive treatment of cancer with minimal side effects. One of the promising approaches is by targeted destruction of cancerous cells using localized heating.

The destruction of tumors by locally heating tissue sufficient to cause its demise has been under investigation for some time. The benefits of thermal therapeutics over conventional removal by surgery are numerous; most thermal approaches are minimally or non-invasive, relatively simple to perform, and have the potential of treating tumors embedded in vital regions where surgical removal is not feasible.

Ideally, the activating energy to heat the tumor would be targeted on the embedded tumor with minimal effect on surrounding healthy tissue.

Unfortunately, conventional heating techniques such as focused ultrasound, microwaves, and laser light do not discriminate between tumors and surrounding healthy tissue.

Thus success has been modest and typically results in some damage to surrounding tissue. Recent work around the world suggests that nanostructures designed to attach to cancerous cells may provide a very powerful means for highly localized energy absorption at the sites of cancerous cells.

Researchers at Rice University in the USA recently reported work on mice in which gold-coated nanoparticles treated to attach to cancerous cells were heated using infrared radiation. Sources of infrared radiation, in a manner analogous to radio stations, can be tuned to transmit at a narrow band of electromagnetic frequencies. Additionally, dimensions of the "nanoshells" can be changed to absorb a particular infrared radiation frequency. Researchers can thereby choose a frequency of the infrared radiation that couples with the gold coated nanoparticles, and at the same time does not couple to the tissue of the body, enabling selective destruction of cancerous cells and tumors.

The results of a carefully controlled experimental trial with mice, while preliminary, were very encouraging. Mice into which cancerous cells were introduced and were treated with the nanoshells-infrared radiation therapy appeared healthy and tumor free more than 90 days later; all those receiving the same introduction of cancerous cells and not treated had their cancers grow to such an extent that they were euthanized after an average of 12 days.

In Europe, work at Charité Hospital in Berlin, coupled with scientists at the Friedrich-Schiller-Universität Jena, have shown that magnetic nanoparticles interstitially injected directly into the tumor-heated with radio-frequency radiation-can destroy cancer cells in a human brain tumor and is also believed to enhance the effects of subsequent radiation therapy. The nanoparticles localize on the tumor due to a special biomolecularly modified outer layer-leaving surrounding health tissue with minimum damage.

SMART AND DYNAMIC NANOPLATFORMS

In Japan work at Nagoya University with magnetite cationic liposomes (MCLs) combined with heat shock proteins has shown great potential in cancer treatment as well. Using the MCLs, the researchers demonstrated that they could locally generate heat in a tumor by placing test mice in an alternating magnetic field and not cause the body temperature of the test animal to rise. Following injection of the MCLs and application of an alternating magnetic field, tumor temperature and body temperature differed by 6ºC. The combined treatment strongly inhibited tumor growth over a 30-day period and complete regression of tumors was observed in 20% of the mice.

This parallel progress in applications of nanotechnology for the treatment of cancer illustrates the global interest in nanoscience and its potential application to innovative medical technologies. Further, the fact that several groups, using related but different techniques, can demonstrate positive results increases the chances that this new approach might be a powerful new approach to the treatment of cancer.

3

Proton Therapy: from Pioneering Work to Clinical Application

What twenty years ago was basic research has now developed into a tumour treatment potentially available in hospitals worldwide. Patients with optical tumours were first given radiation treatment with protons at PSI in the early eighties. Since then, almost 4500 patients have been treated, with convincing results. Under the PROSCAN project PSI has developed a new type of proton accelerator, suitable for use in hospitals. This superconducting cyclotron is used in conjunction with spot-scanning, a special radiation procedure for the treatment of deep-seated tumours.

By using this technique the advantages of protons for cancer treatment, in comparison with conventional radiation therapy using photons, can be fully utilised. Healthy tissue is particularly well protected and it is possible to irradiate very large, complex tumours, where there is no other comparable treatment method. The spot-scanning procedure endows PSI with a leading position worldwide in proton therapy.

Co-operation and licensing contracts have been completed with industrial companies to make it possible for hospitals to acquire the system. Various centres are already under construction, or at the planning stage, and will depend on the expertise of PSI. The PROSCAN project is based on many years of preparatory basic research at PSI in accelerator physics and radiation biology and is an excellent example of how the results of pure scientific curiosity can one day mutate into beneficial applications.

SMALL INTERFERING RNA (SIRNA) TECHNOLOGY

The third approach involves small interfering RNA (siRNA) technology, which is currently emerging as a potentially useful method to develop highly specific double stranded RNA-based gene silencing therapeutic. The aim is to develop efficient and effective siRNA delivery systems for tumors in the central nervous system (Project Co-ordinators: A/P Wang Shu and A/P Sheu Fwu-Shan).

Role of Cellular and Molecular Biomechanics

Cellular and molecular biomechanics of cancer cells can be a fascinating area, which characterizes the rheological properties of mutant cancer cells and relates the measurable mechanical properties to their molecular basis. Changes in the rheological properties may provide useful information for cancer diagnosis and physical evidence to understand therapeutic mechanisms of various anti-cancer agents.

Recent advances in experimental biomechanics have enabled direct and real-time mechanical probing and manipulation of single cells and molecules. Such methods are now capable of imposing and sensing forces and displacements with nano and picoscale resolutions. Experimental Methods and ToolsThe experimental techniques to probe single cells include micropipette aspiration, optical/laser traps and atomic force microscopy. Focus will be made on the original biochemical conditions of the cancerous cells, as well as drug treatment for which the mechanical properties of these cells can either increase or decrease, as compared to the healthy cell. Such changes in mechanical response with the underlying changes in molecular architecture as a consequence of disease development, and how that changes cell shape and mobility, can also be observed.

Research Aims of the Nano Biomechanics Laboratory

Their Nano Biomechanics Laboratory has been well established in the area of nanomechanics of biological cells and molecules. It will focus its effort on investigating biomechanical responses to the progression of the disease state of cancer cells as well as the effects arising from treatment using anti-cancer agents/molecular drugs.

Research Grants Allocated

They have successfully obtained a few research grants from the Singapore Cancer Syndicate (SCS) and BMRC, A*STAR. They shall file more grant applications based on this synergistic program. We shall also contact pharmaceutical companies for industrial investment on this synergistic program. International collaboration with top universities and in the world will be widened and strengthened.

BIODEGRADABLE PARTICLES MIMIC WHITE BLOOD CELLS

Scientists have developed biodegradable polymers that can mimic the ability of white blood cells to target inflamed blood vessel walls, according to a new study led by Ohio University researchers. The finding could be the first step in developing drugs that suppress specific sites of inflammation in medical conditions such as arthritis, heart disease and inflammatory bowel disease.

Researchers found that biodegradable beads coated with targeting molecules can travel through the bloodstream and effectively stick to the site of tissue inflammation, a symptom of various diseases, according to the study, which will be published in the Dec. 23 issue of the journal Proceedings of the National Academy of Sciences. Scientists are interested in drugs made from biodegradable polymers because they can be easily prepared, have a long shelf life and can be designed to release specific doses of medication, according to the study.

When the body suffers from a bacterial infection or a wound, the white blood cells, or leukocytes, adhere to the site to treat the problem. But in inflammatory diseases such as arthritis, heart disease or inflammatory bowel disease, leukocytes accumulate in an area where they aren't needed and cause or progressively worsen the disease.

To address that issue, Ohio University researcher Douglas Goetz and colleagues Justin Hanes of Johns Hopkins University, Kevin Shakesheff of the University of Nottingham in England, Mohammad Kiani of the University of Tennessee Health Science Center and David Kurjiaka of Ohio University have been studying whether biodegradable particles could be used to mimic the activity of leukocytes, traveling to the exact site of the inflammatory disease in the body and delivering treatment. Conventional drugs treat pathological inflammation, but may impact healthy tissue too.

"Can we take a particle and give it the same surface chemistry as the leukocyte and make it go where the leukocyte goes?" asked Goetz, an associate professor of chemical engineering whose research is funded by the National Science Foundation and the Whitaker Foundation.

The new study suggests that in animal models, a biodegradable bead can be coated with targeting molecules and show the same level of adhesion as leukocytes. Shakesheff originally developed the bead, which is made of polylactic acid and polyethylene glycol, two polymers commonly used in other medical applications, Goetz said. This biodegradable particle was 100 times more effective at sticking to the blood vessel wall than other materials tested in previous studies, the engineer said. The bead degrades and converts to lactic acid, a substance normally found in the body. Goetz and colleagues, using novel polymers developed by Hanes, next will test different polymers-as well as smaller nanoparticles-that could degrade even faster in the body and offer different drug delivery options, he said. Quick degradation also could help avoid uptake by organs not intended to receive the particles, he said, a possible negative side effect of the process.

The research team also will further examine another interesting finding from the study: The biodegradable particles not only mimic the leukocyte's ability to stick to tissue, but its tendency to roll along the blood vessel wall. Though Goetz is unsure what impact this finding will have on drug delivery at this point, "it demonstrates how well we can control these particles-not only with selective delivery, but also the type of relationship they have with the vessel wall," he said.

Goetz, who next will study the drug delivery potential for chronic inflammatory conditions, hopes that the combined cell adhesion/drug delivery approach to addressing inflammation-related illnesses will progress in the next 10 years.

Other scientists are making progress in creating a targeted drug delivery process to eradicate cancerous tumors, but applying such concepts to inflammatory diseases will call for some fine-tuning, he said. "Applying this to inflammation is a whole different ball game," Goetz said. "A patient probably won't die from arthritis; it's a much more subtle problem." Other collaborators on the study are Harshad Sakhalkar, an Ohio University graduate student in chemical engineering; Milind Dalal, a former Ohio University graduate student in chemical engineering; Aliasger Salem of the University of Nottingham; Ramin Ansari of the University of Tennessee Health Science Center; and Jie Fu of Johns Hopkins University.

Molecular Labeling Might Improve Cancer Diagnosis

Although there is no thorough cure for cancer at late stage, early stage cancer is treatable in general and the prognosis could be great. Cancer diagnosis is thus an important and practical way to improve the cure rate. The current diagnosis techniques are usually in tissue level, which has low efficiency and fails to detect invisible cancer cells. Molecular imaging has become a high area in cancer diagnosis. Molecular labeling is a key. The existing ways of labeling and visualizing DNA and protein molecules rely on the light-emitting properties of a limited group of radioactive elements, chemical dyes, and protein molecules.

Problems Associated with Labeling Methods

These labeling techniques have several drawbacks: radioactive markers have short life spans, while organic dyes come with a limited number of colors and may quickly lose their glow. There have been great demands for more reliable and more robust labeling fluorophores, to enable real-time imaging and quantitative determination of multiple-molecule types present in cells.

Advantages of Using Quantum Dots in Medical Imaging and Labeling

Highly luminescent quantum dots can overcome the functional limitations encountered with chemical and organic dyes. They are highly stable against photo-bleaching and have narrow, symmetric emission spectra. In particular, the emission wavelength of quantum dots can be continuously tuned by changing the particle size or composition, and a single light source can be used for simultaneous excitation of all different-colored dots.

Aims of this Nanobiotechnology Cancer Research Project

This synergistic program will develop robust biological nanoprobes using optically active quantum dots for multi-parameter and quantitative analysis of genes and proteins in tissues.

This research will include synthesis of high quality luminescent quantum dots, a reasonable understanding of the surface chemistry for bioconjugation, and the preparation of water-soluble and biocompatible nanocrystals for real-time monitoring, simultaneous screening and quantitative bio-imaging of multiple biochemical contents in cancerous organisms by using confocal micro-spectrophotometer. The research will be focused more on cancer diagnosis.

Nanosensors for Cancer Detection

Another technology which will be developed in this synergistic program is nanosensors. Sensors constructed at the molecular scale are promising and have achieved to be extremely sensitive, selective and responsive, which can be used to replace more costly and tedious laboratory methods for monitoring a patient's blood for proteins, chemicals and pathogens.

This FG has utilized high-density well-aligned carbon nanotubes, which are multi-walled and vertically aligned on a large area of substrates. They have a unique expertise in developing electrochemical multiwalled nanotubes, ordered nanotube arrays, chemically functionalized nanotubes, and conjugated polymers as nanosensors.

Developing Lab-on-a-Chip Devices

This synergistic program in near future will develop two fully integrated laboratory-on-a-chip devices for cancer diagnosis. The first contains numerous functional features such as indicators for physical parameters and reaction chambers for cell growth and separation at micro-and nano-scale to rapid identify cancer cells.

Potential cancer cells can be delivered into the microfluidic device and possibly cultivated in-vitro followed by detection using various optical-based detection methods.

Building Beads-Based Lab-on-a-Chip Device

The second is a beads-based lab-on-chip device to rapidly identify metabolites, genes and singlenucleotide-polymorphism (SNP) sites associated with specific cancers. The two lab-on-chip devices have several distinct advantages over the current cell culturing and detection methods, which include ease of use for cell culture and reaction, rapid hybridization and sensitive detection, and low cost for commercial interest.

Currently Used Methods for Treating Cancer

The standard treatment for cancer has been surgery plus radiotherapy in the past decades. If cancer patients fail such a treatment, he/she has only less than 10% to be cured by other treatment such as chemotherapy, immunotherapy, and molecular therapy. Chemotherapy is one of the most effective treatments available for cancer and other diseases such as cardiovascular diseases and AIDS. The present status of chemotherapy, however, is far from being satisfactory. Its efficacy is limited and patients have to suffer from severe side effects.

Nanobiotechnology is Solving Problems Associated with Chemotherapy Treatments?

Nanobiotechnology may provide an ideal solution for the problems in the current regime of chemotherapy and promote a new concept of chemotherapy, which may include sustained, controlled and targeted chemotherapy; personalized chemotherapy; chemotherapy across various physiological drug barriers such the gastrointestinal (GI) barrier for oral chemotherapy and the blood-brain barrier (BBB) for treatment of brain tumors and other central nerve system (CNS) diseases; and eventually, chemotherapy at home.

Nanobiotechnology may Change the Way That Drugs are Made

Indeed nanobiotechnology, especially nanoparticle technology, will change the way we make drugs and the way we take drugs. Paclitaxel, one of the best antineoplastic drugs found from nature in the past decades, will be used as a prototype drug in this synergistic program due to its excellent therapeutic efficacy against a wide spectrum of cancers, and its great commercial success as one of the best sellers among various antineoplastic agents.

Our preliminary results have shown by fluorescence microscopy and cell mortality experiment with HT-29 cells that paclitaxel formulated by Vitamin E TPGS-emulsified PLGA nanoparticles can be at least 18 times more effective than the free drug Taxol® after 24 hours of cell culture, and oral chemotherapy by nanoparticles seems feasible.

Other Cancer Research Areas that this Project Will Explore

We shall continue to be focused on our established strength which includes synthesis of co-polymers more friendly to anti-cancer drugs and molecular drugs (proteins and peptides), characterization and application of natural emulsifiers such as phospholipids, cholesterols and molecularly modified vitamins, surface medication techniques, enhanced molecular conjugation techniques and nanoparticle techniques. Our research will speed up to animal test and clinical trials.

Gene Therapy, Targeted Gene Delivery and Gene Transfer

Gene therapy will also be a focus of this synergistic program. Targeted gene delivery to selected cell types provides a means for highly specific gene expression. Improved efficiency of gene transfer could be achieved through enhancing the entry of gene vectors into the desired cells and reducing the uptake of the vectors by non-target cells.

Developing Materials for Research

We are developing chimeric peptides, containing a nucleic acid binding domain linked to a receptor-binding domain of neurotrophins, to target gene delivery vectors to tumor cells. These and other functional peptides are also tried to be conjugated to cationic polymer-based DNA vectors. The developed materials would hopefully form stable nanoparticles with DNA that are suitable for in vivo targeting of cancer gene therapy.

What is a Cell-Specific Promoter and How Does It Work?

The second approach is to use a cell-specific promoter in a viral vector, which allows the control of specific gene expression in a selected cell type. Because of their cellular authentic sequences, the cell-specific promoter may reduce the chance of activating host cell defense machinery and are usually less sensitive to cytokine-induced promoter inactivation than viral promoters, thus improving the stability of gene expression.

REMOTELY ACTIVATED NANOPARTICLES DESTROY CANCER CELLS

The first in a new generation of nanotechnology-based cancer treatments will likely begin clinical trials in 2007, and if the promise of animal trials carries through to human trials, these treatments will transform cancer therapy. By replacing surgery and conventional chemotherapy with noninvasive treatments targeted at cancerous tumors, this nanotech approach could reduce or eliminate side effects by avoiding damage to healthy tissue. It could also make it possible to destroy tumors that are inoperable or won't respond to current treatment.

One of these new approaches places gold-coated nanoparticles, called nanoshells, inside tumors and then heats them with infrared light until the cancer cells die. Because the nanoparticles also scatter light, they could be used to image tumors as well. Mauro Ferrari, a leader in the field of nanomedicine and professor of bioengineering at the University of Texas Health Science Center, says this is "very exciting" technology. "With chemotherapy," Ferrari says, "we carpet bomb the patient, hoping to hit the lesions, the little foci of disease. To be able to shine the light only where you want this thing to heat up is a great advantage."

Although several groups are now working on similar localized treatments, Naomi Halas and Jennifer West have led the way in this area, and their work is the farthest along. (See "Nano Weapons Join the Fight Against Cancer.") Nearly ten years ago, Halas, professor of chemistry and electrical and computer engineering at Rice University, developed a precise and reliable method for making nanoshells, which can be hollow spheres of gold or, in the case of the cancer treatment, gold-coated glass spheres. These spheres are small enough (about 100 nanometers in diameter) to slip through gaps in blood vessels that feed tumors. So as they circulate in the bloodstream, they gradually accumulate at tumor sites.

Halas tuned the nanoparticles to absorb specific wavelengths of light by changing the thickness of the glass and gold. For the cancer treatment, she selected infrared wavelengths that pass easily through biological tissues without causing damage. To destroy a nanoshell-infiltrated tumor, the tumor is illuminated with a laser, either through the skin or via an optical fiber for areas such as the lungs.

"We shine light through the skin, and in just a few minutes, the tumor is heated up," Halas says. "In the studies that were initially reported--and this has been repeated now more than 20 times in at least three different animal models--we have seen essentially 100 percent tumor remission." The tests also suggest the nanoshells are nontoxic. Halas says they are eliminated from the body through the liver over several weeks. The technology was developed at Rice in collaboration with Jennifer West, a professor of bioengineering. It has been licensed by Nanospectra Biosciences, a startup based in Houston, TX, that is beginning the process of getting FDA approval for clinical trials for treating head and neck cancer. In the future, the technology could be used for a wide variety of cancers.

"There is a potential for this to bring a profound change in cancer treatment," Halas says. "For the case of someone discovering a lump in their breast, this would mean that a very simple procedure could be performed that would induce remission." She says that "for many, many cases of cancer, rather than the lengthy chemotherapy or radiation therapy," an individual would have "one simple treatment and very little side effects."

Halas anticipates that approval for the method will come quickly, in part because the nanotechnology is not a drug but a device, for which the approval process is simpler. Also, she expects it will perform the same in humans as in animal models, "because heat and light work in exactly the same way whether you're in a pig, a dog, [or] a human being."

Since their initial experiments, the researchers have been further developing the technology. They've demonstrated the ability to coat the nanoshells with antibodies that latch on to breast-cancer cells, further improving the selectivity of the treatment. They've also attached molecules that make the nanoshells into pH sensors that would be useful for both imaging tumors and as an "optical biopsy" for identifying cancers, Halas says.

The clinical trials this year will not take advantage of these advances. But eventually the antibody targeting could make preventative cancer treatments possible. "If you have the genetic profile for prostate cancer occurring in your family, one could imagine treating extremely early stages, when you have something a millimeter or smaller which you could barely visualize," Halas says. "With antibody targeting and then illumination of that region, you could destroy those cells at a very early stage. You could have a treatment every five to ten years, and then you would be free of the disease." The nanotechnology could also be used to eradicate cancers that have spread too much to be removed by surgery. While people will not be able to take advantage of these advances in the near future, Halas says that treatments based on the original design could be available in a couple of years. Ferrari cautions that most treatments do not make it through clinical trials, but, he says, "I'm hopeful that their clinical trials will yield great results."

KNOWING DISEASE BEFORE IT BEGINS

Nanotechnology may one day help physicians detect the very earliest stages of serious diseases like cancer, a new study suggests. It would do so by improving the quality of images produced by one of the most common diagnostic tools used in doctors' offices â€" the ultrasound machine.

In laboratory experiments on mice, scientists found that nano-sized particles injected into the animals improved the resulting images. This study is one of the first reports showing that ultrasound can detect these tiny particles when they are inside the body, said Thomas Rosol, a study co-author and dean of the college of veterinary medicine at Ohio State University.

"Given their tiny size, nobody thought it would be possible for ultrasound to detect nanoparticles," he said. It turns out that not only can ultrasound waves sense nanoparticles, but the particles can brighten the resulting image. One day, those bright spots may indicate that a few cells in the area may be on the verge of mutating and growing out of control.

"The long-term goal is to use this technology to improve our ability to identify very early cancers and other diseases," said Jun Liu, a study co-author and an assistant professor of biomedical engineering at Ohio State University. "We ultimately want to identify disease at its cellular level, at its very earliest stage." The study is in the current issue of the journal Physics in Medicine and Biology. The researchers injected a solution of silica nanoparticles into the tail vein of each mouse. They then anesthetized the animals and placed them on their backs on a warm imaging table.

Rosol said that Liu and her team are working on creating biodegradable nanoparticles. For the purposes of this study, however, the researchers wanted to use a hard substance, silica, to see if their idea would work. The strongest ultrasound signals are those produced by sound waves bounce off a hard surface. While not biodegradable, the nanoparticles used in the study were biologically inert.

The researchers took ultrasound images of the animals' livers every five minutes for 90 minutes after the injection. The nanoparticles had accumulated in the animals' livers. Another future step for this work is to label nanoparticles with a molecular road map of sorts, which would direct the particles to go to specific locations in the body.

"The liver takes up foreign substances in the body, so it's not surprising that that's where we saw the particles," Rosol said. "But we ultimately want to be able to make these particles to go to the mammary glands or other tissues we're interested in." The ultrasound images grew brighter over the 90-minute period. The researchers compared these images to those from a group of control mice injected with a saline solution. There was no change in ultrasound image brightness in the control mice after that injection. While this research is still in its infancy, Rosol and his colleagues foresee a day when nanotechnology can alert a physician to the beginnings of cancer or heart disease, perhaps in a woman who has a family history of breast cancer: "Her doctor could inject the breast with nanoparticles and the resulting ultrasound image would alert the doctor to any suspicious areas in the tissue, even at the cellular level," Rosol said.

The hope is that combining ultrasound and nanotechnology may provide a definitive diagnosis in lieu of an invasive procedure like a biopsy. "These nanoparticles may make it possible for physicians to screen for tumors very quickly, and perhaps lessen the need for a biopsy in many cases," Liu said. Nanoparticles are smaller than any cell in the human body, so they may pass through the walls of the leaky blood vessels, or capillaries, of tumor tissue and actually infiltrate the tumor.

"Until now, nobody knew what these particles would do in the blood," Rosol said. "But they made it into the liver. And despite their miniscule size, nanoparticles are still big enough to carry a payload of medicine," Rosol said. "That the particles made it into the liver suggests that they could be used to deliver toxic chemotherapeutic drugs that would act locally on a tissue, at the site of a tumor, and not have such a pronounced affect on the rest of the body," Rosol said. "The problem with chemotherapy is that the drug affects the whole body, causing a host of problems such as hair loss, diarrhea and anemia."

EARLIER DETECTION

The University of South Florida was awarded $8 million by state officials to create the Florida Center of Excellence for Biomolecular Identification and Targeted Therapeutics. The state award will be combined with $39 million from the City of Tampa, Hillsborough County, Florida High Tech Corridor Council, and USF for a total investment of $47 million to create a center that will develop technologies to respond to and treat biological threats and then translate these technologies info commercial products which will benefit the environment and public health. Also involved is Biovest International, a Worchester, MA, biotech company that hopes to cooperate on research and development efforts with the new USF center. USF projects that the return on investment to the region includes creation of 400 new biotechnology jobs, $84 million in direct wages and an estimated economic impact of over $188 million.

Earlier detection, targeted cancer therapy focus of nanotechnology collaboration between Moffitt, USF.

By 2020 it is projected there will be 16.5 million new cancer cases, 3.8 million in the United States, according to the World Health Organization. With such a global concern, researchers and the medical society are turning to the littlest details, sweating the smallest stuff and finding exceptional potential with nanotechnology. H. Lee Moffitt Cancer Center & Research Institute, the University of South Florida College of Medicine and the USF Nanomaterials and Nanomanufacturing Research Center (NNRC) have been collaborating for several years to develop and apply nanotechnology to treating cancer. On December 8, the collaboration will host the region's first conference on nanotechnology advances in disease detection and therapy. Open to the public, this conference will feature local and national experts in the field, including Dr. Robert Blumenthal from the National Cancer Institute and Nanobiosym, Inc. Founder, Dr. Anita Goel. The program will begin at 8 a.m. at the Vincent A. Stabile Research building at Moffitt.

APPLICATIONS OF NANOTECHNOLOGY TOOLS AND PRODUCTS

The applications of nanotechnology are extremely diverse, mainly because the field is interdisciplinary. In addition, the effect that nanotechnology will have during the next decade is difficult to estimate because of potentially new and unanticipated applications. For example, if simply reducing the microstructure in existing materials can make a big market impact, then this may, in turn, lead to a whole new set of applications. However, it seems reasonable to assume that during the next two to three years most activity in nanotechnology will still be in the area of research, rather than completed projects or products.

Moving from Research to the Market

Holister estimates that there are currently 455 public and private companies, 95 investors, and 271 academic institutions and government entities that are involved in the near-term applications of nanotechnology worldwide. The ability of such institutions to transfer research results into industrial applications can be indicated by the number of filed patents. Compano and Hullman provide an analysis of this, using the number of nanopatents filed at the European Patent Office (EPO) in Munich. Over the whole 1981-1998 period, the number of nanopatents rises from 28-180 patents, with an average growth rate in the 1990s amounting to 7%.

PHOTOLITHOGRAPHY WORLD RECORDS

Progress in micro-electronics leads to ever-faster and ever-cheaper products, and is based on the production of ever-smaller electrical circuits. Photolithography is the critical production step whereby these tiny circuits are "printed" on silicon chips. Against the background of this technological trend, research is being carried out into the ongoing development of lithography techniques at the Swiss Light Source (SLS) of PSI. The newly-operational XIL beamline uses light in the extreme ultraviolet (EUV) range in order to make very small patterns in photoresist-films. During 2004, researchers succeeded in using this technique to produce structures with periods of 32 nanometres, which corresponds to a line width as small as 16 nm. This represents the highest resolution achieved so far in recording images using photons-a world record! The structures made at the SLS are used in diverse research fields, including the development of EUV lithography technology for the fabrication of future computer chips, magnetic data storage media and X-ray optics.

MICRO MAGNETISM

Very small magnetic particles have areas where the magnetic needles of all the atoms point in the same direction. Synchrotron light makes these domains visible, and lets us investigate their reaction to applied magnetic fields. Although people have known about magnetism for over 3000 years, we still have no theory to explain why some materials are magnetic and some are not. A new experiment at the Swiss Light Source (SLS) enables us to see the orientation of magnetic fields in particles of just a few thousandths of a millimetre in diameter. The SLS, which is one of the most modern synchrotrons in the world, provides the extremely short and bright pulses of X-ray light necessary for such exacting research. The investigation into magnetic domains looks at the changes that happen when an external magnetic field is applied to the domains. This provides information about the forces acting between the magnetic needles of the atoms. The results of this work are of great interest for basic research, but they also have important technical applications. For example, very small magnetic particles store information on computer hard discs.

NEW EXPLORATIONS

Most scientists agree that nanorobots will not be developed for many years, if ever. Instead, current research in nanotechnology is focused on nanomaterials, tiny particles of organic and inorganic matter.

These particles and their potential uses in the treatment of cancer are being investigated at The University of Texas M. D. Anderson Cancer Center. Specifically, researchers are looking at ways in which nanomaterials might be used to deliver targeted treatments to cancer cells.

Nanotechnology refers to materials, devices, and systems created through the manipulation of matter on a nanometric scale and the exploitation of novel phenomena and properties that occurs at that scale. At 1/80,000th the width of a human hair, a nanometer is the length of 10 hydrogen atoms placed end to end. The possible applications of nanotechnology are innumerable, but medicine and computer science are expected to be among the first fields to yield viable products and techniques. Nanotechnology is already in use in a few commercially available products, including sunscreen and wrinkle-free pants.

Nanomaterials are created using either a "top-down" or "bottom-up" approach. The top-down approach refers to etching and molding materials into smaller and smaller components and is applicable to computer technology, whereas the bottom-up approach involves assembling structures atom by atom or molecule by molecule and is therefore more suited to medical research.

Gravity exerts control over such things as an ant, a person, or a red dwarf star. However, material smaller than a nanometer is governed not by gravity but by the laws of quantum mechanics. Nanomaterials exist between these two worlds, resulting in odd but exploitable behavior. "Nanotechnology is kind of a test-tube wonder in search of an application," said Michael G. Rosenblum, Ph.D., a professor in the Department of Bioimmunotherapy at M. D. Anderson.

Working with such small materials in medicine poses unique problems. Nanoparticles are so small that they can be cleared out of the body before they complete their mission. They also have large surface areas relative to their volumes, which allows for easier manipulation but means that friction can be a problem.

Specialized nanoparticles called nanoshells are the focus of a research collaboration between John D. Hazle, Ph.D., chair (ad interim) and associate professor in the Department of Imaging Physics at M. D. Anderson, and engineers at Rice University in Houston.

Nanoshells, which are hollow spheres made of silica and sometimes coated with gold, were invented by Naomi Halas, Ph.D., a professor of electrical and computer engineering and chemistry at Rice University.

Antibodies can be attached to the surface of nanoshells, causing the shells to target certain cells. Laser light directed onto the shells from outside of the body would cause them to superheat, destroying tumor cells but leaving healthy cells unaffected.

This application of nanoshells is especially attractive in the treatment of prostate cancer; the prostate is near the surface of the body and therefore more easily accessible than other tumor sites. "You could theoretically spare most of the gland and just kill the part of the gland that has the tumor cells," said Dr. Hazle.

Coating the shells with gold has distinct advantages; gold colloids have been used in medicine for years and are known to have low toxicity. "It's very inert, but you can also do the chemistry needed to bind antibodies and other biomolecules to the gold. These nanoshells can mimic gold colloids; the body doesn't know that they're shells instead of particles," said Dr. Hazle.

Dr. Hazle expects that the use of gold nanoshells in tumor ablation will enter clinical trials in three to four years. "What we're focusing on is the best way to target cells and get them in a high enough concentration to either directly damage all of the surrounding tumor cells with heat or coagulate the microvasculature and starve them [the tumor cells] though a lack of blood and oxygen," he said.

Nanoshells also could be filled with a drug-containing polymer. Heating the shells would cause the polymer to change shape, squeezing out a controlled amount of the drug.

"The shells that were activated would either burst or become permeable enough that the drugs would be able to escape into the local environment, so you could do more of a locoregional therapy and get a much higher local tissue concentration of a drug than you would be able to get systemically," said Dr. Hazle.

Physicians have no way to accurately control the release rate of time-release drug implants, and patients who need regular doses of a medication must go to the doctor's office often to have the drug administered. Using drug-filled nanoshells would allow for a more accurate rate of drug release and for patients to release the drug themselves by heating the implanted particles with an infrared light.

Dr. Rosenblum is studying another type of chemotherapeutic drug delivery system by applying nanotechnology's most famous discovery, buckminsterfullerene, or the buckyball. A nanoparticle composed of 60 carbon atoms in the shape of a soccer ball, the buckyball earned its discoverers, Sir Harold W. Kroto, Ph.D., of the University of Sussex, UK, and Robert F. Curl, Jr., Ph.D., and Richard E. Smalley, Ph.D., both of Rice University, the 1996 Nobel Prize in Chemistry.

"We're trying to put chemotherapeutic agents on the surface of these particles so that they will be active when they are delivered to the target cell," said Dr. Rosenblum.

The current method of attaching drugs directly to antibodies has not been successful because each element in the pair adversely affects the other. A buckyball could carry separately the drug and the antibodies needed to target a particular cell. It also could deliver more than one kind of drug simultaneously.

"What these particles will allow us to do is to link these drugs together on the surface of the sphere in a combination that is synergistic, hopefully delivering that combination punch to the target cell with our antibodies," said Dr. Rosenblum.

Dr. Rosenblum's group is also evaluating whether buckyballs can safely and efficiently deliver radioisotopes to cancer cells. Calculations suggest that, in most cases, the radioisotopes will not escape their carbon cages before they reach the cells. Buckyballs could potentially deliver currently unusable radioisotopes, such as radon and actinium-225, to tumor cells. "It has the potential for holding radioisotopes for which there is no known chelator, that is, no way to link these isotopes to carrier molecules," said Dr. Rosenblum.

Research into these techniques is still confined to the laboratory and, according to Dr. Rosenblum, there is no way to predict when they might be tested in clinical trials. "Before we do it, there's no way of knowing how it is going to work," he said. "We don't even know what the challenges are at this point, but all of the things we are going to find out are going to be new; that's the interesting part."

Nano 'Tinkertoys' may Improve Cancer Therapy

U-M researchers have developed a faster, more efficient way to produce a wide variety of nanoparticle drug delivery systems, using DNA molecules to bind the particles together. Nanometer-scaled dendrimers can be assembled in many configurations by using attached lengths of single-stranded DNA molecules, which naturally bind to other DNA strands in a highly specific fashion.

"With this approach, you can target a wide variety of molecules-drugs, contrast agents-to almost any cell," says Dr. James R. Baker Jr., the Ruth Dow Doan Professor of Nanotechnology and director of the Center for Biologic Nanotechnology.

Nanoparticle complexes specifically can be targeted to cancer cells and are small enough to enter a diseased cell, either killing it from within or sending out a signal to identify it. But making the particles is notoriously difficult and time-consuming.

The nanoparticle system used by Baker's lab is based on dendrimers, star-like synthetic polymers that can carry a vast array of molecules on the ends of their arms.

It is possible to build a single dendrimer carrying many different kinds of molecules such as contrast agents and drugs, but the synthesis process is long and difficult, requiring months for each new molecule added to the dendrimer in sequential steps. And the yield of useful particles drops with each successive step of synthesis.

For a paper published Jan. 21 in the journal Chemistry and Biology, Biomedical Engineering graduate student Youngseon Choi built nanoparticle clusters of two different functional dendrimers, one designed for imaging and the other for targeting cancer cells. Each of the dendrimers also carried a single-stranded, non-coding DNA synthesized by Choi.

In a solution of two different kinds of single dendrimers, these dangling lengths of DNA-typically 34-66 bases long-found complementary sequences on other dendrimers and knitted together, forming barbell shaped two-dendrimer complexes with folate on one end and fluorescence on the other end.

Folate receptors are over-expressed on the surface of cancer cells, so these dendrimer clusters would tend to flock to the diseased cells. The other end of the complex carries a fluorescent protein so that the researchers can track their movement.

A series of experiments using cell sorters, 3-D microscopes and other tools verified that these dendrimers hit their targets, were admitted into the cells and gave off their signaling light. The self-assembled dendrimer clusters were shown to be well formed and functional.

"This is the proof-of-concept experiment," Choi says. But now that the assembly system has been worked out, other forms of dendrimer clusters are in the works.

"If you wanted to make a therapeutic that targeted five drugs to five different cells, it would be 25 synthesis steps the traditional way," Baker says. "At two to three months per synthesis, and a significant loss of yield for each step, that approach just wouldn't be practical."

Instead, the Baker group will create a library of single-functional dendrimers that can be synthesized in parallel, rather than sequentially, and then linked together in many different combinations with the DNA strands. "So it's like having a shelf full of Tinkertoys," Baker says.

An array of single-functional dendrimers, such as targets, drugs and contrast agents, and the ability to link them together quickly and easily in many different ways would enable a clinic to offer 25 different "flavors" of dendrimer with only 10 synthesis steps, Baker says.

Baker foresees a nanoparticle cluster in which a single dendrimer carries three single-strands of DNA, each with a sequence specific to the DNA attached to other kinds of dendrimers. Put into solution with these other tinker toys, the molecule would self-assemble into a four-dendrimer complex carrying one drug, one target and one fluorescent.

'Nanospice' as a novel nanotechnology strategy for human cancer therapy

(Nanowerk News) Curcumin, a yellow polyphenol extracted from the rhizome of turmeric (Curcuma longa), has potent anti-cancer properties as demonstrated in a plethora of human cancer cell line and animal carcinogenesis models. Nevertheless, widespread clinical application of this relatively efficacious agent in cancer and other diseases has been limited due to poor aqueous solubility, and consequently, minimal systemic bioavailability. Nanotechnology drug delivery approaches have the potential for rendering hydrophobic agents like curcumin dispersible in aqueous media, thus circumventing the pitfalls of poor solubility.

A group of researchers in India have synthesized a polymeric nanoparticle encapsulated formulation of curcumin-nanocurcumin-utilizing the micellar aggregates of cross-linked and random copolymers of N-isopropylacrylamide (NIPAAM), with N-vinyl-2-pyrrolidone (VP) and poly (ethyleneglycol) monoacrylate (PEG-A). ("Polymeric nanoparticle-encapsulated curcumin (nanocurcumin): a novel strategy for human cancer therapy"-free access article) Nanocurcumin, unlike free curcumin, is readily dispersed in aqueous media. Nanocurcumin demonstrates comparable in vitro therapeutic efficacy to free curcumin against a panel of human pancreatic cancer cell lines, as assessed by cell viability and clonogenicity assays in soft agar.

Further, nanocurcumin's mechanisms of action on pancreatic cancer cells mirror that of free curcumin, including induction of cellular apoptosis, blockade of nuclear factor kappa B (NFkappaB) activation, and downregulation of steady state levels of multiple pro-inflammatory cytokines (IL-6, IL-8, and TNFalpha). Nanocurcumin provides an opportunity to expand the clinical repertoire of this efficacious agent by enabling ready aqueous dispersion. Future studies utilizing nanocurcumin are warranted in pre-clinical in vivo models of cancer and other diseases that might benefit from the effects of curcumin.

4

Nanomaterials and Micro/Nano-Sized Devices for Cancer Therapy

Currently, nanomaterials are in the leading position (in comparison to futuristic nanotechnologies e.g., surgical nanomachines) in terms of extensive research, application and products in pipeline.

The nanomaterials have the inherent advantage of possessing unique functional properties for cancer detection and treatment. Certain nanomaterials such as gold nanoparticles have the advantage to be manufactured in large quantities and hence are more cost-effective. Nanomaterials get classified in the size domain of proteins and cells. Hence they have been used as biological tags by interfacing the nanoparticles with biocompatible molecules (biological, small organic molecules or bio-inorganic interface).

The shape and dimensions of nanomaterials can be altered to obtain special capabilities, such as cellular membrane penetration. Size distribution plays a critical role, when the nanoparticles are engineered to exhibit their specialized physical properties such as optical absorbance and fluorescence.

In contrast to nanomaterials for biomarker applications, specially engineered biomolecules have been developed (e.g., hairpin-shaped oligonucleotides), which consists of a fluorophore and quencher moiety. The oligonucleotides behave like switches, where if they undergo conformational changes by intermolecular interactions, the hairpin structure is opened separating the quencher and fluorophore moiety resulting in fluorescence.

In spite of the superior advantage of such engineered biomolecules, they currently face a challenge to strike a balance between cost-effectiveness and performance reliability. The reports of cancer diagnostics and therapeutics based on nanomaterials research and upcoming products are in pipeline.

MEANING AND DEFINITION

Nanotechnology, popularly known as the science of small or scientifically described as the technology to develop materials and structures of the size range from 1 to 100 nanometres.

Oncologists all over the globe, relentlessly research on methodologies for early detection of cancer and precise localization of cancer therapeutics (radiation/chemotherapy) with minimal adverse effects to healthy tissues. Since the previous decade, the fast growing research in nanotechnology has shown promising possibilities for achieving this dream of every oncologist.

Since three to four years certain research efforts have been transformed into nanotech based products in pipeline (undergoing clinical trials) in early detection of cancer detection and cancer therapeutics.

The aim of this review is provide the reader about both, the futuristic prospects of currently pursued cancer nanotechnology research and practical innovations arising out of successful research projects. The second half of the review consists of discussion on nanotech products in pipeline. In addition, various other interdisciplinary engineering marvels with potential of significant impact in cancer nanotechnology, have been mentioned in brief.

NANOMATERIAL TECHNOLOGY

Nanomaterial-based catalysts are usually heterogeneous catalysts broken up into nanoparticles in order to speed up the catalytic process. The extremely small size of the particles maximizes the surface area exposed to the reactant, allowing more reactions to occur at the same time, thus speeding up the process. Much research on nanomaterial-based catalysts have to do with maximizing the effectiveness of the catalyst coating in fuel cells. Platinum is currently the most common catalyst for this application, however, it is expensive and rare, so a lot of research has been going into maximizing the catalytic properties of other metals by shrinking them to nanoparticles in the hope that someday they will be an efficient and economic alternative to platinum.

Defense programs in many countries are now concentrating on nanotechnology research that will facilitate advances in such technology used to create secure but small messaging equipment, allow the development of smart weapons, improve stealth capabilities, aid in developing specialized sensors (including bio-inclusive sensors), help to create self-repairing military equipment, and improve the development and delivery mechanisms for medicines and vaccines. Nanotechnology builds on advances in microelectronics during the last decades of the twentieth century. The miniaturization of electrical components greatly increased the utility and portability of computers, imaging equipment, microphones, and other electronics. Indeed, the production and wide use of such commonplace devices such as personal computers and cell phones was absolutely dependent on advances in microtechnology.

Despite these fundamental advances there remain real physical constraints (e.g., microchip design limitations) to further miniaturization based upon conventional engineering principles. Nanotechnologies intend to revolutionize components and manufacturing techniques to overcome these fundamental limitations. In addition, there are classes of biosensors and feedback control devices that require nanotechnology because-despite advances in microtechnology-present components remain too large or slow.

ADVANCES

Nanotechnology advances affect all branches of engineering and science that deal directly with device components ranging in size between 1/10,000,000 (one ten millionth of a millimeter) and 1/10,0000 millimeter. At these scales, even the most sophisticated microtechnology-based instrumentation is useless. Engineers anticipate that advances in nanotechnology will allow the direct manipulation of molecules in biological samples (e.g., proteins or nucleic acids) paving the way for the development of new materials that have a biological component or that can provide a biological interface.

In addition to new tools, nanotechnology programs advance practical understanding of quantum physics. The internalization of quantum concepts is a necessary component of nanotechnology research programs because the laws of classical physics (e.g., classical mechanics or generalized gas laws) do not always apply to the atomic and near-atomic level. Nanotechnology and quantum physics. Quantum theory and mechanics describe the relationship between energy and matter on the atomic and subatomic scale. At the beginning of the twentieth century, German physicist Maxwell Planck (1858-1947) proposed that atoms absorb or emit electromagnetic radiation in bundles of energy termed quanta. This quantum concept seemed counter-intuitive to well-established Newtonian physics. Advancements associated with quantum mechanics (e.g., the uncertainty principle) also had profound implications with regard to the philosophical scientific arguments regarding the limitations of human knowledge.

Planck's quantum theory, which also asserted that the energy of light (a photon) was directly proportional to its frequency, proved a powerful concept that accounted for a wide range of physical phenomena. Planck's constant relates the energy of a photon with the frequency of light. Along with the constant for the speed of light, Planck's constant (h = 6.626 x 10-34 Joule-second) is a fundamental constant of nature.

Prior to Planck's work, electromagnetic radiation (light) was thought to travel in waves with an infinite number of available frequencies and wavelengths. Planck's work focused on attempting to explain the limited spectrum of light emitted by hot objects. Danish physicist Niels Bohr (1885-1962) studied Planck's quantum theory of radiation and worked in England with physicists J. J. Thomson (1856-1940), and Ernest Rutherford (1871-1937) to improve their classical models of the atom by incorporating quantum theory. During this time, Bohr developed his model of atomic structure.

According to the Bohr model, when an electron is excited by energy it jumps from its ground state to an excited state (i.e., a higher energy orbital). The excited atom can then emit energy only in certain (quantized) amounts as its electrons jump back to lower energy orbits located closer to the nucleus. This excess energy is emitted in quanta of electromagnetic radiation (photons of light) that have exactly the same energy as the difference in energy between the orbits jumped by the electron.

The electron quantum leaps between orbits proposed by the Bohr model accounted for Plank's observations that atoms emit or absorb electromagnetic radiation in quanta. Bohr's model also explained many important properties of the photoelectric effect described by Albert Einstein (1879-1955). Einstein assumed that light was transmitted as a stream of particles termed photons. By extending the well-known wave properties of light to include a treatment of light as a stream of photons, Einstein was able to explain the photoelectric effect. Photoelectric properties are key to regulation of many microtechnology and proposed nanotechnology level systems.

Quantum mechanics ultimately replaced electron "orbitals" of earlier atomic models with allowable values for angular momentum (angular velocity multiplied by mass) and depicted electron positions in terms of probability "clouds" and regions.

In the 1920s, the concept of quantization and its application to physical phenomena was further advanced by more mathematically complex models based on the work of the French physicist Louis Victor de Broglie (1892-1987) and Austrian physicist Erwin Schrödinger (1887-1961) that depicted the particle and wave nature of electrons. De Broglie showed that the electron was not merely a particle but a waveform. This proposal led Schrödinger to publish his wave equation in 1926. Schrödinger's work described electrons as a "standing wave" surrounding the nucleus, and his system of quantum mechanics is called wave mechanics. German physicist Max Born (1882-1970) and English physicist P. A. M. Dirac (1902-1984) made further advances in defining the subatomic particles (principally the electron) as a wave rather than as a particle and in reconciling portions of quantum theory with relativity theory.

Working at about the same time, German physicist Werner Heisenberg (1901-1976) formulated the first complete and self-consistent theory of quantum mechanics.

Matrix mathematics was well established by the 1920s, and Heisenberg applied this powerful tool to quantum mechanics. In 1926, Heisenberg put forward his uncertainty principle which states that two complementary properties of a system, such as position and momentum, can never both be known exactly.

This proposition helped cement the dual nature of particles (e.g., light can be described as having both wave and particle characteristics). Electromagnetic radiation (one region of the spectrum that comprises visible light) is now understood to have both particle and wave like properties.

In 1925, Austrian-born physicist Wolfgang Pauli (1900-1958) published the Pauli exclusion principle states that no two electrons in an atom can simultaneously occupy the same quantum state (i.e., energy state). Pauli's specification of spin (+1/2 or-1/2) on an electron gave the two electrons in any suborbital differing quantum numbers (a system used to describe the quantum state) and made completely understandable the structure of the periodic table in terms of electron configurations (i.e., the energy-related arrangement of electrons in energy shells and suborbitals).

In 1931, American chemist Linus Pauling published a paper that used quantum mechanics to explain how two electrons, from two different atoms, are shared to make a covalent bond between the two atoms. Pauling's work provided the connection needed in order to fully apply the new quantum theory to chemical reactions.

Advances in nanotechnology depend upon an understanding and application of these fundamental quantum principles. At the quantum level the smoothness of classical physics disappears and nanotechnologies are predicated on exploiting this quantum roughness.

NANOTECHNOLOGY: THE NEXT LEAP

While the physicist-led team at U. Brob was finishing its work on the AFM-based molecular manipulator, a chemist-led team at the University of

Lilliput was working furiously. They saw the U. Brob desktop machine as too large and its expected products as too expensive. Even back in the 1980s, David Biegelsen of the Xerox Palo Alto Research Center had noted, "The main drawback I see to using a hybrid protoassembler [AFM-based molecular manipulator] is that it would take a long time to build just one unit. Building requires a series of atom-by-atom construction steps. It would be better to build in parallel from the very beginning, making many trillions of these molecules all at the same time. I think there is tremendous power in parallel assembly. Maybe another field, chemistry or biology, offers a better way to do it." The chemists at U. Lill aimed to develop that better way, building first simple and then more and more complex molecular machines. The eventual result was a primitive molecular assembler able to build molecular objects by the trillions.

Chemist's Tools

How did the chemists achieve this? During the years when the U. Brob team was developing the molecular manipulator, researchers working in protein science and synthetic chemistry had made better and better systems of molecular building blocks. Chemists were well prepared for doing this: by the late 1980s, it had become possible to build stable structures the size of medium-sized protein molecules, and work had begun to focus on making these molecules perform useful work by binding and modifying other molecules. Chemists learned to use these sophisticated catalysts-early molecular devices-to make their own work easier by helping in the manufacture of still more large molecules.

Another traditional chemist's tool was software for doing computer-aided design. The early software designed by Jay Ponder and Frederic Richards of Yale University ultimately led to semi-automatic tools for designing molecules of a particular shape and function. Chemists then could easily design molecules that would self-assemble into larger structures, several tens of nanometers across.

MOLECULAR CONSTRUCTION MACHINES

These advances in software and chemical synthesis let the U. Lill team tackle the task of building a primitive version of a molecular assembler. Although they couldn't build anything as complex as a nanocomputer or as stiff as diamond, they didn't need to. Their design used sliding molecular rods to position a molecular gripper much like the gripper used at U. Brob, again using the surrounding liquid to control which tool the gripper held. Instead of an AFM's electronic controls, they used the surrounding liquid to control the position of the rods as well. In a neutral solution, the rods would withdraw; in an acid solution, they would extend. How far they moved depended on what other molecules were around to lodge in special pockets and block the motion.

Their primitive assemblers built much the same sorts of products that the U. Brob molecular manipulator did; the tools were similar, and speed and accuracy were about the same. Yet there was one dramatic advantage: About 1,000,000,000,000,000,000,000 U. Lill assemblers could fit in the space occupied by one U. Brob manipulator, and it was easy to produce a mere 1,000,000,000,000,000 times as much product at the same cost.

With the first, primitive assemblers, construction was slow because each step required new liquid baths and several seconds of soaking and waiting, and a typical product might take thousands of steps.

Nonetheless, the U. Lill team made a lot of money licensing their technology to researchers trying to commercialize products they had first researched with the U. Brob machine. After starting an independent company (Nanofabricators, Inc.), they poured their research efforts into building better machines.

Within a few years, they had assemblers with multiple grippers, each loaded with a different kind of tool; flashes of colored light would flip molecules from state to state (they copied these molecules from the pigments of the retina of the eye); flipping molecules would change tools and change rod positions.

Soaking and waiting become a thing of the past, and soon they were pouring out parts that, when mixed with liquid and added to dishes with special blank chips would build up the dense memory layers that made possible the Pocket Library.

That was when things started moving fast. The semiconductor industry went the way of the vacuum tube industry. Money and talent poured into the new technology.

Molecular CAD tools got better, assemblers made it easy to build what was designed, and fast production and testing made molecular engineering as easy as playing with software. Assemblers got better, faster, and cheaper. Researchers used assemblers to build nanocomputers, and nanocomputers to control better, faster assemblers. Using tools to build better tools is an ancient story. Within a decade, almost anything could be made by molecular manufacturing, and was.

PROPERTIES OF NANOMATERIALS

In tandem with surface-area effects, quantum effects can begin to dominate the properties of matter as size is reduced to the nanoscale. These can affect the optical, electrical and magnetic behaviour of materials, particularly as the structure or particle size approaches the smaller end of the nanoscale. Materials that exploit these effects include quantum dots, and quantum well lasers for optoelectronics.

For other materials such as crystalline solids, as the size of their structural components decreases, there is much greater interface area within the material; this can greatly affect both mechanical and electrical properties. For example, most metals are made up of small crystalline grains; the boundaries between the grain slow down or arrest the propagation of defects when the material is stressed, thus giving it strength. If these grains can be made very small, or even nanoscale in size, the interface area within the material greatly increases, which enhances its strength. For example, nanocrystalline nickel is as strong as hardened steel. Understanding surfaces and interfaces is a key challenge for those working on nanomaterials, and one where new imaging and analysis instruments are vital.

NANOMATERIAL SCIENCE

Nanomaterials are not simply another step in the miniaturization of materials. They often require very different production approaches. There are several processes to create nanomaterials, classified as 'top-down' and 'bottom-up'. Although many nanomaterials are currently at the laboratory stage of manufacture, a few of them are being commercialised. Below we outline some examples of nanomaterials and the range of nanoscience that is aimed at understanding their properties. As will be seen, the behaviour of some nanomaterials is well understood, whereas others present greater challenges.

APPLICATIONS OF NANOMATERIALS

Below we list some key current and potential shortand long-term applications of nanomaterials. Most current applications represent evolutionary developments of existing technologies: for example, the reduction in size of electronics devices.

Current Applications

Nanosized titanium dioxide and zinc oxide are currently used in some sunscreens, as they absorb and reflect ultraviolet (UV) rays and yet are transparent to visible light and so are more appealing to the consumer. Nanosized iron oxide is present in some lipsticks as a pigment but it is our understanding that it is not used by the European cosmetics sector. The use of nanoparticles in cosmetics has raised a number of concerns about consumer safety.

Composites

An important use of nanoparticles and nanotubes is in composites, materials that combine one or more separate components and which are designed to exhibit overall the best properties of each component. This multifunctionality applies not only to mechanical properties, but extends to optical, electrical and magnetic ones. Currently, carbon fibres and bundles of multiwalled CNTs are used in polymers to control or enhance conductivity, with applications such as antistatic packaging.

The use of individual CNTs in composites is a potential long-term application. A particular type of nanocomposite is where nanoparticles act as fillers in a matrix; for example, carbon black used as a filler to reinforce car tyres. However, particles of carbon black can range from tens to hundreds of nanometres in size, so not all carbon black falls within our definition of nanoparticles.

Clays

Clays containing naturally occurring nanoparticles have long been important as construction materials and are undergoing continuous improvement. Clay particle based composites – containing plastics and nanosized flakes of clay – are also finding applications such as use in car bumpers.

Coatings and Surfaces

Coatings with thickness controlled at the nano- or atomic scale have been in routine production for some time, for example in molecular beam epitaxy or metal oxide chemical vapor depositionfor optoelectonic devices, or in catalytically active and chemically functionalized surfaces.

Recently developed applications include the self-cleaning window, which is coated in highly activated titanium dioxide, engineered to be highly hydrophobic (water repellent) and antibacterial, and coatings based on nanoparticulate oxides that catalytically destroy chemical agents.

Wear and scratch-resistant hard coatings are significantly improved by nanoscale intermediate layers (or multilayers) between the hard outer layer and the substrate material.

The intermediate layers give good bonding and graded matching of elastic and thermal properties, thus improving adhesion.

A range of enhanced textiles, such as breathable, waterproof and stainresistant fabrics, have been enabled by the improved control of porosity at the nanoscale and surface roughness in a variety of polymers and inorganics.

Tougher and Harder Cutting Tools

Cutting tools made of nanocrystalline materials, such as tungsten carbide, tantalum carbide and titanium carbide, are more wear and erosion-resistant, and last longer than their conventional (large-grained) counterparts. They are finding applications in the drills used to bore holes in circuit boards.

Short-term Applications

Paints

Incorporating nanoparticles in paints could improve their performance, for example by making them lighter and giving them different properties. Thinner paint coatings ('lightweighting'), used for example on aircraft, would reduce their weight, which could be beneficial to the environment. However, the whole life cycle of the aircraft needs to be considered before overall benefits can be claimed. It may also be possible to substantially reduce solvent content of paints, with resulting environmental benefits. New types of foulingresistant marine paint could be developed and are urgently needed as alternatives to tributyl tin (TBT), now that the ecological impacts of TBT have been recognised.

Anti-fouling surface treatment is also valuable in process applications such as heat exchange, where it could lead to energy savings. If they can be produced at sufficiently low cost, fouling-resistant coatings could be used in routine duties such as piping for domestic and industrial water systems. It remains speculation whether very effective anti-fouling coatings could reduce the use of biocides, including chlorine. Other novel, and more long-term, applications for nanoparticles might lie in paints that change colour in response to change in temperature or chemical environment, or paints that have reduced infra-red absorptivity and so reduce heat loss.

Concerns about the health and environmental impacts of nanoparticles may require the need for the durability and abrasion behaviour of nano-engineered paints and coatings to be addressed, so that abrasion products take the form of coarse or microscopic agglomerates rather than individual nanoparticles.

Remediation

The potential of nanoparticles to react with pollutants in soil and groundwater and transform them into harmless compounds is being researched. In one pilot study the large surface area and high surface reactivity of iron nanoparticles were exploited to transform chlorinated hydrocarbons (some of which are believed to be carcinogens) into less harmful end products in groundwater. It is also hoped that they could be used to transform heavy metals such as lead and mercury from bioavailable forms into insoluble forms. Serious concerns have been raised over the uncontrolled release of nanoparticles into the environment.

Fuel Cells

Engineered surfaces are essential in fuel cells, where the external surface properties and the pore structure affect performance. The hydrogen used as the immediate fuel in fuel cells may be generated from hydrocarbons by catalytic reforming, usually in a reactor module associated directly with the fuel cell. The potential use of nano-engineered membranes to intensify catalytic processes could enable higher-efficiency, small-scale fuel cells. These could act as distributed sources of electrical power. It may eventually be possible to produce hydrogen locally from sources other than hydrocarbons, which are the feedstocks of current attention.

Displays

The huge market for large area, high brightness, flat-panel displays, as used in television screens and computer monitors, is driving the development of some nanomaterials.

Nanocrystalline zinc selenide, zinc sulphide, cadmium sulphide and lead telluride synthesized by sol–gel techniques (a process for making ceramic and glass materials, involving the transition from a liquid 'sol' phase to a solid 'gel' phase) are candidates for the next generation of light-emitting phosphors. CNTs are being investigated for low voltage field-emission displays; their strength, sharpness, conductivity and inertness make them potentially very efficient and long-lasting emitters.

Batteries

With the growth in portable electronic equipment (mobile phones, navigation devices, laptop computers, remote sensors), there is great demand for lightweight, high-energy density batteries. Nanocrystalline materials synthesized by sol–gel techniques are candidates for separator plates in batteries because of their foam-like (aerogel) structure, which can hold considerably more energy than conventional ones. Nickel–metal hydride batteries made of nanocrystalline nickel and metal hydrides are envisioned to require less frequent recharging and to last longer because of their large grain boundary (surface) area.

Fuel Additives

Research is underway into the addition of nanoparticulate ceria (cerium oxide) to diesel fuel to improve fuel economy by reducing the degradation of fuel consumption over time.

Catalysts

In general, nanoparticles have a high surface area, and hence provide higher catalytic activity. Nanotechnologies are enabling changes in the degree of control in the production of nanoparticles, and the support structure on which they reside. It is possible to synthesise metal nanoparticles in solution in the presence of a surfactant to form highly ordered monodisperse films of the catalyst nanoparticles on a surface. This allows more uniformity in the size and chemical structure of the catalyst, which in turn leads to greater catalytic activity and the production of fewer byproducts.

It may also be possible to engineer specific or selective activity. These more active and durable catalysts could find early application in cleaning up waste streams. This will be particularly beneficial if it reduces the demand for platinum-group metals, whose use in standard catalytic units is starting to emerge as a problem, given the limited availability of these metals.

Longer-term Applications

CNTs have exceptional mechanical properties, particularly high tensile strength and light weight. An obvious area of application would be in nanotubereinforced composites, with performance beyond current carbon-fibre composites. One current limit to the introduction of CNTs in composites is the problem of structuring the tangle of nanotubes in a well-ordered manner so that use can be made of their strength. Another challenge is generating strong bonding between CNTs and the matrix, to give good overall composite performance and retention during wear or erosion of composites.

The surfaces of CNTs are smooth and relatively unreactive, and so tend to slip through the matrix when it is stressed. One approach that is being explored to prevent this slippage is the attachment of chemical side-groups to CNTs, effectively to form 'anchors'. Another limiting factor is the cost of production of CNTs. However, the potential benefits of such light, high strength material in numerous applications for transportation are such that significant further research is likely.

Lubricants

Nanospheres of inorganic materials could be used as lubricants, in essence by acting as nanosized 'ball bearings'. The controlled shape is claimed to make them more durable than conventional solid lubricants and wear additives. Whether the increased financial and resource cost of producing them is offset by the longer service life of lubricants and parts remains to be investigated. It is also claimed that these nanoparticles reduce friction between metal surfaces, particularly at high normal loads. If so, they should find their first applications in high-performance engines and drivers; this could include the energy sector as well as transport. There is a further claim that this type of lubricant is effective even if the metal surfaces are not highly smooth. Again, the benefits of reduced cost and resource input for machining must be compared against production of nanolubricants. In all these applications, the particles would be dispersed in a conventional liquid lubricant; design of the lubricant system must therefore include measures to contain and manage waste.

Magnetic Materials

It has been shown that magnets made of nanocrystalline yttrium–samarium–cobalt grains possess unusual magnetic properties due to their extremely large grain interface area (high coercivity can be obtained because magnetization flips cannot easily propagate past the grain boundaries).

This could lead to applications in motors, analytical instruments like magnetic resonance imaging (MRI), used widely in hospitals, and microsensors. Overall magnetisation, however, is currently limited by the ability to align the grains' direction of magnetisation. Nanoscale-fabricated magnetic materials also have applications in data storage.

Devices such as computer hard disks depend on the ability to magnetize small areas of a spinning disk to record information.

If the area required to record one piece of information can be shrunk in the nanoscale (and can be written and read reliably), the storage capacity of the disk can be improved dramatically. In the future, the devices on computer chips which currently operate using flows of electrons could use the magnetic properties of these electrons, called spin, with numerous advantages. Recent advances in novel magnetic materials and their nanofabrication are encouraging in this respect.

Medical Implants

Current medical implants, such as orthopaedic implants and heart valves, are made of titanium and stainless steel alloys, primarily because they are biocompatible. Unfortunately, in some cases these metal alloys may wear out within the lifetime of the patient. Nanocrystalline zirconium oxide (zirconia) is hard, wearresistant, bio-corrosion resistant and bio-compatible. It therefore presents an attractive alternative material for implants. It and other nanoceramics can also be made as strong, light aerogels by sol–gel techniques. Nanocrystalline silicon carbide is a candidate material for artificial heart valves primarily because of its low weight, high strength and inertness.

Machinable Ceramics

Ceramics are hard, brittle and difficult to machine. However, with a reduction in grain size to the nanoscale, ceramic ductility can be increased. Zirconia, normally a hard, brittle ceramic, has even been rendered superplastic (for example, able to be deformed up to 300% of its original length). Nanocrystalline ceramics, such as silicon nitride and silicon carbide, have been used in such automotive applications as high-strength springs, ball bearings and valve lifters, because they can be easily formed and machined, as well as exhibiting excellent chemical and high-temperature properties. They are also used as components in high-temperature furnaces. Nanocrystalline ceramics can be pressed into complex net shapes and sintered at significantly lower temperatures than conventional ceramics.

Water Purification

Nano-engineered membranes could potentially lead to more energy-efficient water purification processes, notably in desalination by reverse osmosis. Again, these applications would represent incremental improvements in technologies that are already available. They would use fixed nanoparticles, and are therefore distinct from applications that propose to use free nanoparticles.

Military Battle Suits

Enhanced nanomaterials form the basis of a state-of- the-art 'battle suit' that is being developed by the Institute of Soldier Nanotechnologies at MIT. A short-term development is likely to be energy-absorbing materials that will withstand blast waves; longer-term are those that incorporate sensors to detect or respond to chemical and biological weapons (for example, responsive nanopores that 'close' upon detection of a biological agent). There is speculation that developments could include materials which monitor physiology while a soldier is still on the battlefield, and uniforms with potential medical applications, such as splints for broken bones.

DIFFERENT ROLES PLAYED BY NANOTECHNOLOGY

Much of todays Nano scale research is designed to reach a better understanding of how matter behaves on this small scale. The factors that govern larger systems do not necessarily apply on the Nano scale. Because Nano materials have large surface areas relative to their volumes, phenomena like friction and sticking are more important than they are in larger systems.

NANO-BASICS

Nanotechnology in Nature

Living organisms are examples of Natures handy work of Nanotechnology, many natural molecular machines systems display enormous abilities. Molecular machinery in green plants converts more energy and synthesizes a greater tonnage of organic compounds than a chemical industry, and does it job so cleanly using cheap raw materials picked up by itself. The storage capacity of genome in few bacteria may far exceed that in any large computer systems of today. Nature places far denser systems in the same volume free of charge (no-technical sophistication and resources spent up).

Natural molecular machinery has outperformed anything we now know, how to build. There is lot to learn from nature about building molecular machines of our own design, aiming to make a wider range of products, including computer components that we can actually put to use.

Molecular Machine Systems

Photo courtesy NASA, Ames Nanogears no more than a nanometer wide could be used to construct a matter compiler, which could be fed raw material to arrange atoms and build a macro-scale structure.

If something has moving parts and does useful work, we call it a machine. If something is nanometers in scale and has a precise arrangement of bonded atoms, we call it a molecule, or a molecular assembly. If something matches both these descriptions, we can properly call it a molecular machine; if it comprises many parts, each worthy of the name 'machine', it may be better described as molecular machine system.

Manufactured products are made from atoms. The properties of those products depend on how those atoms are arranged. Viewed from the molecular level today's macroscopic manufacturing methods are crude and imprecise. Casting, milling, welding and all the other traditional manufacturing methods spray atoms about in great statistical herds. Even lithography (which already lets us put millions of transistors on a chip no bigger than your fingernail) is fundamentally statistical and random. Exactly how many dopant atoms are in a single transistor and exactly where each individual dopant atom is located is neither specified nor known: if we have roughly the right number in roughly the right place, we can make a working transistor. For today, that is good enough.

The exception is chemistry. Large high purity crystals can have almost every atom in the right place. So, too, can many long polymers. The structures of proteins with hundreds and even thousands of amino acids can be specified down to the last atom. Most dramatically (and fortunately for us!) DNA strands with many tens of millions of bases can be copied with almost perfect accuracy. And it seems that almost any small molecule (with perhaps several dozens of atoms) can be synthesized, if only we have the skill and patience. Yet the laws of physics and chemistry in principle permit arranging and rearranging the elements in so many combinations and permutations that all of our manufacturing skills and all of our chemical skills barely suffice to scratch the surface of what is possible. Such descriptions don't define sharp boundaries. Although it seems hard not to view the bacterial flagellar motor as a molecular machine, somewhere on the path towards simplicity--from ribosome to enzyme, organ metallic catalyst, or solvated ion-the term 'machine' loses its utility.

A straightforward analysis based on well-established physical principles shows that these advanced devices can process matter, energy, and information precisely, efficiently, and with high productivity. Theoretical studies have explored synthetic strategies for such structures, guiding reactions by atomically precise positioning of highly reactive species. These synthetic strategies, however, themselves rely on preexisting molecular machinery to do the positioning. Concrete progress in Nanotechnology can be achieved from the existing conventional technologies. Since the most attractive approaches involve solvated, self-assembled systems of folded macromolecules, it should come as no surprise that biotechnology and allied fields are well positioned to exploit them at the earliest possible opportunity.

Elaboration of this principle in more difficult directions has led to the design and synthesis of branched, three-dimensional structures, including a cube-like framework containing eight Y junctions, and a growing range of successors. This work indicates that nucleic acids can be engineered to serve as scaffolding for complex molecular systems. For constructing any machine we require suitable tools to old and place the component in the precise location. The complexity of the tool increases as the size of the component decreases. Imagine a building a component consisting of few molecules-What tools can be used, how they would look like? And How to use them? Development of the right tools for Nanotechnology itself should be a interesting issue. Regardless of whether specifically biological molecules remain the preferred choice for implementing design concepts, ongoing advances in tools for biotechnology will boost molecular machine research. The growth of combinatorial chemistry has strengthened the drive toward high-throughput, automated systems for chemical synthesis and analysis. Improved microfluidic systems--'labs on a chip'--will make experiments faster and cheaper, expanding the utility of trial and error in overcoming limited predictive knowledge and design methods. Micromechanical systems in the form of scanning probe microscopes now enable direct visualization and manipulation of individual macromolecules.

Biomimetic System

Nature chiefly relies on proteins and nucleic acids for molecular machine components, but evolution has responded to different incentives that differ from ours, and been locked into the same basic chemistry for billions of years. By learning from nature and then applying the tools of organic synthesis to realize quite different designs, we can gain still more freedom to avoid problems and implement solutions.

Biomimetic Machinery

With computational modeling to aid rational design, and faster, cheaper cycles of synthesis and analysis to correct mistakes, it seems that emerging technologies will eventually enable the routine fabrication of diverse macromolecular objects comparable in function to proteins. Since proteins in nature form molecular machine systems, it seems worth considering what analogous systems could do for us. Manufactured products are made from atoms. The properties of those products depend on how those atoms are arranged. If we rearrange the atoms in coal we can make diamond. If we rearrange the atoms in sand (and add a few other trace elements) we can make computer chips. If we rearrange the atoms in dirt, water and air we can make potatoes. Todays manufacturing methods are very crude at the molecular level. Casting, grinding, milling and even lithography move atoms in great thundering statistical herds. In the future, It will be possible to snap together the fundmental building blocks of nature easily, inexpensively and in most of the ways permitted by the laws of physics. This will be essential if we are to continue the revolution in computer hardware beyond the next decade, and will also let us fabricate an entire new generation of products that are cleaner, stronger, lighter, and more precise. It's worth pointing out that the word "nanotechnology" has become very popular and is used to describe many types of research where the characteristic dimensions are less than about 1,000 nanometers. For example, continued improvements in lithography have resulted in line widths that are less than one micron: this work is often called "nanotechnology." Sub-micron lithography is clearly very valuable in electronics

Common Structures used in Nanotechnology

Nanotube are the most common structures used in Nano technology. Nanotubes are made of carbon atoms bonded into honeycomb-like shapes with enormous strength and electrical conductivity. Recently another structure made of different oxides is Nano belt. Nano belt manufacturing seems to be simpler and produces belts which are longer than Nanotubes. Nanopores is another structure the pores are so small that DNA separation is being attempted using this structure. Quantum dots are minuscule molecule making up tiny crystals that glow when stimulated by ultraviolet light. Nanoshells are miniscule beads coated with gold. Dendrimers are man-made molecules about the size of an average protein, and have a branching shape. As the research in the field progress, more structures would be identified.

Nanoshells

Nanoshells are miniscule beads coated with gold. By manipulating the thickness of the layers making up the nanoshells, scientists can design these beads to absorb specific wavelengths of light. The most useful nanoshells are those that absorb near-infrared light, which can easily penetrate several centimeters of human tissue. The absorption of light by the nanoshells creates an intense heat that is lethal to cells.

Dendrimers

Research is being done on a number of Nano particles created to facilitate drug delivery. One such molecule with potential to link treatment with detection and diagnosis is known as a dendrimer. Dendrimers are man-made molecules about the size of an average protein, and have a branching shape. This shape gives them vast amounts of surface area to which scientists can attach therapeutic agents or other biologically active molecules. Researchers aim eventually to create nanodevices that do much more than deliver treatment.

Nanotechnologies in Patient Care

Nanotechnologies that will aid in cancer care are in various stages of discovery and development. Experts believe that quantum dots, nanopores, and other devices for detection and diagnosis may be available for clinical use in five to 15 years. Therapeutic agents are expected to be available within a similar time frame. Devices that integrate detection and therapy could be used clinically in about 15 or 20 years. Nanotech could affect medicine, industry, and the fabrication of just about everything you buy, because smaller is not just beautiful, but also cheaper, faster and less wasteful of energy.

Nanobelts may turn out to have advantages over tubes in terms of price, flexibility and practicality. For making Nanobelts oxide is evaporated for two hours, what the researchers called "white woollike products" appeared on a plate in a cooler part of the furnace. Using electron microscopes and X-ray diffraction, Wang and his crew analyzed that itty-bitty woolly stuff. Nanobelt is deposited as woollike product. The oxide contained zinc, tin, cadmium, gallium or indium, the little straps have a rectangular cross-section, with a width of 30 to 300 nanometers and a thickness of 10 to 15 nanometers. Because the material is already an oxide, it does not undergo a chemical reaction, and has a pure, flawless surface.

More important, each belt was a single crystal. Flawlessness is a big advantage, says Wang, professor of material science and engineering and director of Georgia Technology's Center for Nano science and Nano technology. He attributes the lack of flaws to the minuscule size. "They are so small that no defect can stay in the volume, they just pop out." While Nano tubes are generally only a few millionths of a meter long, the belts are millimeters long. And while Nano tubes are made of pure carbon, belts have already been made from five oxides, a much greater variety for the engineer to play with. "The oxide world is so colorful, so fancy," says Wang, "but carbon is only carbon." Nanodevices as a link between detection, diagnosis, and treatment. Researchers aim eventually to create nanodevices that do much more than deliver treatment. The goal is to create a single nanodevice that will do many things: assist in imaging inside the body, recognize precancerous or cancerous cells, release a drug that targets only those cells, and report back on the effectiveness of the treatment.

Sensors: The electrical conductivity of zinc oxide, for example, changes drastically when a gas molecule attaches, so zinc oxide is already used to detect flammable gases. Tiny sensors could replace existing ones, and find new uses as well.

Smart Windows: These high-tech pieces of glass respond to temperature changes by, for example, restricting the flow of ultraviolet light. Tin oxide treated with fluoride is currently used for this purpose.

Flat-panel Displays: Indium oxide doped with tin is transparent, but electrically conducting, making it a promising material for advanced displays.

Electronic and Optical-electronic Devices: The tested oxides are semiconductors and are the main members of the "smart and functional materials" family. Thus nanobelts could be used to make tiny devices for electronic or fiber-optics purposes. The worlds economy is largely based on defense need of the countries. Huge amount is spent in procurement, development, manufacture and maintaining equipment. The lower price due to nanotechnology would reduce budget for defense, space exploration. Newer eco friendly material for building construction could provide more energy efficient and comfortable housing. Nano device could also help better and cheaper management of waste generated in the cities.

BUILDING WITH MOLECULAR GRIPPERS AND TOOLS

To build something with the U. Brob team's AFM-based molecular manipulator system, you use it as follows: First, choose a surface to build on and place it under the tip in a pool of liquid. Then dunk the AFM tip into the liquid, bringing it down to the surface, and back it off a little. Construction can now begin as soon as a tool is loaded into the gripper.

Tubes and pumps can flow different liquids over the surface and past the gripper, carrying different tool molecules. If you want to do something with a tool of Type A, you wash in the proper liquid. Once it is in the gripper, you can use the AFM mechanism to move it around and put it where you want it. Move it up to the surface at a convenient spot, wait a few seconds, and it reacts, forming a bond and leaving a molecular fragment attached to the spot you chose. To add a different fragment, you can use a tool of Type B: you back up the tip, flow in a fresh liquid carrying the new tools, and in a moment a tool of the new type is bound in place and ready to apply, either on or alongside the first spot. Step by step, you build up a precise molecular structure.

Each step takes only seconds. Molecular tools pop into the gripper in a fraction of a second, and used tools pop off at the same rate. Once the tip has positioned a molecule, it reacts quickly, about a million times faster than unwanted reactions at other sites. In this way, the molecular manipulator gives good control of where reactions will occur (though it is not as reliable as an advanced assembler would be). It is fairly fast by a chemist's standards—per cycle—but still a million times slower than an advanced assembler. It can perform a variety of steps, but isn't as flexible and capable as an advanced assembler. In short, it is hardly the last word in nanotechnology, yet is a great advance over what has gone before.

Products

With its ability to accelerate desired reactions by a factor of a million or so, the U. Brob team's molecular manipulator can perform 10,000 to 100,000 steps with good reliability. Back in the 1980s, chemists making protein molecules struggled to perform just one hundred steps. The U. Brob research team (and its many imitators) can now build structures that are stronger and easier to design than proteins: not floppy, folded chains, but rugged objects held together by a sturdy network of bonds. Though not as strong and dense as diamond, these structures are like bits of a tough engineering plastic. A specially adapted computer-aided design system makes it easy to design molecular objects made from these materials.

Yet the AFM-based molecular manipulator has one grave disadvantage: It does chemistry one molecule at a time, and it ties up a machine as expensive as a car for hours or days to produce that one large molecule. Some molecules, though, are valuable enough to be worth building even one at a time. These draw prompt attention.

A single molecule isn't much use as a dye, a drug, or a floor wax, but it can have substantial value if it provides useful information. The U. Brob team quickly publishes a pile of scientific papers based on experiments with single molecules: they build a molecule, probe it, report the results, and build another. Some of these results show chemists elsewhere in the multibillion-dollar chemical industry how to design new catalysts, molecules that can help make other molecules more cheaply, cleanly, and efficiently. This information is worth a lot.

Three new products of special interest are among the first to be made. The first—molecular electronics—begins with experiments conducted by a research group at a computer chip company. They use their molecular manipulator to build single molecules and probe them, gradually learning how to build the parts needed for molecular electronic computers. These new computers don't immediately become practical, because the costs are too high for making such large molecules with AFM-based technology. Yet some companies begin to produce simpler molecular electronic devices for use in sensors and specialized high-speed signal processing. A specialty industry is born and begins to expand. The second product is a gene reader, a complex molecular device built on the surface of a chip. The biologists who built the reader combined proteins borrowed from cells with special-purpose molecular machines designed from scratch. The result was a molecular system that binds DNA molecules and pulls them past a read-head-like tape through a tape recorder. The device works as fast as some naturally occurring molecular machines that read DNA, with one key advantage: it outputs its data electronically. At that speed, a single device can read a human genome in about a year. Though still too expensive for a doctor's office, these readers are promptly in great demand from research laboratories. Another small industry is born.

The third product is far more important, in the long run: replacement tips for molecular manipulators, grippers, and tools that are better than the originals. With these new, more versatile devices, researchers are now building more ambitious products and tools.

NANOMATERIALS IN CANCER DETECTION AND IMAGING OF MALIGNANT TISSUES

The optical detection technique (Fluorescence and UV-vis absorption methods) is the most commonly used technique to detect presence of cancer and image cancer tissues with the assistance of biomarker or functionalized nanomaterials; where nanoparticles should either fluoresce or change their optical properties, when they bind to cancer-affected tissues such as silica nanoparticles doped with organic-based fluorescent dyes for detection of liver cell malignancy.

Colloidal CdSe/ZnS-semiconductor nanocrystals (better known as quantum dots) due to their unique physical and photochemical properties have been widely used in in-vivo and in-vitro biological experiments.

Larabell et al, utilized quantum dots for conducting cell motility assay and realized the potential of quantum dots to study cell-signaling events involved in migration and differentiate between invasive and noninvasive cancer cell lines. In addition, Escude et al have used the fluorescence signals from multicolored quantum dots for studying the position and orientation of individual DNA molecules. This methodology can be used to study the variation and existence of oncogenes.

The quantum dots have been incorporated into cationic liposomes for intracellular labeling and imaging applications. Akiyoshi et al, have developed such hybrid nanoparticles to study cancer affected cells at a intracellular level in order to screen various chemotherapeutic candidates and understand their pharmacology.

Due to in-depth research conducted on the optical properties of quantum dots, scientists have modified these properties for providing near infra-red florescence for sentinel lymph node mapping. This technique helped in improvised tracing and identification of affected lymph nodes and significantly reduced pain and the cost of pathology tests required. In addition, there was a significant decrease in major side-effects of breast cancer surgery during routine lymph node removal in breast cancer patients.

Even with new advents in novel nanomaterials, medical professionals all over the globe, still prefer to use nanoparticulate formulation of conventionally used magnetic and paramagnetic materialsdue to its long associated clinical familiarity with the medical professional and well-established performance in both MRI imaging and mapping of malignant tissues. There have been successful attempts where nano-sized and multifunctional particles of iron oxide and gadolinium (G6) compounds have been developed by conjugating them with additional chemical entities and/or materials to make them multifunctional.

Kobayashi and co-workers have used nano-sized formulation of G6 for studying lymphatic drainage by MRI imaging for understanding the metastases of breast cancer. Similarly Fukumori et al have encapsulated gadolinium in chitosan nanoparticles for neuron capture therapy of cancer.

Zhang et al, had succeeded in developing a "nanoprobe" consisting of PEG (Polyethylene Glyocol)-coated iron oxide nanoparticles further functionalized with chlorotoxin and near IR fluorescing molecule Cy5.5. These nanoprobes had preferential uptake in glioma cells and were used for real-time imaging and correlation of preoperative images with intraoperative pathology of gliomas at cellular-level resolution.

Novel Functional Nanomaterials for Cancer Therapy: The advent of nanotechnology in cancer therapy, commenced when diagnostic, chemotherapeutic, antiangiogenesis and gene therapy agents (Engineered Oligonucleotides), were incorporated into nano-sized particles or encapsulation within nano-sized vesicles.

The advantage of sub micron-sized particles (nanometer range and below one micron) is longer duration of circulation time and sustained drug release for improved therapeutic index and reduced toxicity. But time and again scientists and clinicians had to face many challenges of maintaining the therapeutic performance of such novel nano-sized formulations.

There are certain exceptions, where micron-sized drug formulations were proven to be more effective than its nano-sized counterpart. A good example would be the poly(lactic-co-glycolic acid) (PLGA)-methoxy Polyethylene Glycol (mPEG) nanoparticles of cisplatin developed by Avgoustakis et al, which demonstrated a prolonged cisplatin residence in systemic blood circulation, during its clinical studies. The nano-sized formulation possessed the drawback of decreased loading efficiency for therapeutic applications.

Later, scientists and clinicians researched on various encapsulation methods of degradable starch microspheres in an aqueous crystal suspension to intensify intra-arterial chemotherapy of head and neck cancer with high-dose cisplatin.

Subsequently another new method of chemoembolization was established to eliminate drawbacks of previous formulation methods and permitted the usage of low drug doses. Because of early occlusion of the small head and neck vessels and danger of local damage. The biodegradable 6-carboxylcellulose polymer (cisplatin-depot) has also been used in patients with glioblastoma multiforme.

Using innovative chemical engineering techniques, CritiTech Inc. have developed proprietary method of Precipitation with Compressed Antisolvent using supercritical carbon dioxide for pilot plant scale and large scale manufacturability of sub-micron nanoparticles of Paclitaxel. This novel formulation has exhibited promising results of increased survival of tumor-bearing mice to 180 days in comparison to 105 days of tumor-bearing mice treated with regular Paclitaxel formulated with Cremophor. This innovation named as Nanotax, is undergoing Phase 1 clinical trials, for ovarian and pancreatic cancer, which would be administered by intraperitoneal route. Dabur India has a similar formulation undergoing phase III trails (personal communication).

The recent report published in Nature by Sasisekaran et al where his team developed "nanocells" targeted to malignant tissues, is considered to be one of the most innovative multi-functional and intelligent drug delivery methods. This "nanocell" has an outer envelope to be absorbed by the tumor cell and to release an anti-angiogenesis agent for shutdown of blood supply to the tumor and inner nanoparticle release chemotherapeutic agent. This integrative approach to cancer therapy also reduces the drawbacks of receiving decreased therapeutic concentration of chemotherapeutic agent by antiangiogenesis and the increased tumour invasiveness and resistance to chemotherapy caused by over expression of (HIF1-alpha). Other similar innovations include specially specifically engineered nanovectors for tumor-specific gene delivery.

The advent of novel cancer therapeutics from nanotechnology has slowly evolved from nanoencapsulated drug formulations to nano-sized functional nanoparticles. Such functional nanoparticles are engineered to ensure delivery of ionizing radiation, chemotherapeutic agents or thermal dose specifically to malignant tissues.

Most of these functional nanomaterials (nonradioactive in nature) have been used in hyperthermia. Composite metal nanoshells, have been one of the few earliest candidates for infra-red hyperthermia. The dimensions of the nanoshells can be altered to provide optical resonance, which can systematically varied from near-UV to the mid-infrared.

While biocompatible and target specific superparamagnetic and fine ferrimagnetic particles such as Fe_3O_4, have successfully demonstrated hyperthermia by inducing heat under the influence of a strong alternating magnetic field. In addition, improvised success rate was observed in the case of magnetic fluid (ferrofluid) hyperthermia, where magnetic nanoparticles are incorporated in a carrier liquid to easily perfuse in targeted tissues.

PSivida a nanotech company has initiated the Phase II trials of its product "BrachySil" for patients with liver and pancreatic malignancies.

Nanoparticles of silicon impregnated with the radioactive isotope of phosphorus P.BrachySil is injected directly into the cancer using a fine gauge needle. Later, the silicon breaks down and gets excreted. P, which has a half-life of 14 days, eventually decomposes to stable isotopes or is excreted. Because the treatment is localized, the side effects are likely to be less than other forms of brachytherapy.

Gold Nanoparticles: A multifaceted nanomaterial for cancer therapy. Popularly known as colloidal gold and nanogold. The multifaceted abilities of gold have been investigated in-depth right from electronics industry to medicinal formulations of both modern and traditional practices. This multifaceted aspect of gold nanoparticles hasbeen successfully demonstrated in both diagnostics and treatment of cancer.

Compared to many previously mentioned nanomaterials, the synthesis of gold nanoparticles is much simpler and also pose minimal toxicity to kidney and liver, where it accumulates after entering in the systemic circulation.

Optical properties of nanogold is based on the surface plasmon resonance, has been harnessed to provide photodynamic therapy of malignant tissues. Using short laser pulses focused on monoclonal antibodies conjugated with light-absorbing microparticles and nanoparticles. Pitsillides and co-workers reported a improvised methodology for selective cell targeting and providing highly localized cell damage by photodynamic therapy. The method is closely related to chromophore-assisted laser inactivation (involving singlet oxygen) and photodynamic therapy, with an exception of photochemical intermediates. Similar reports have been published on gold nanoparticles and gold coated nanoparticles using infra-red electromagnetic radiation.

Nanogold has shown to have 600 times more absorption in cancer cells than normal human cells. This and the optical property of nanogold to absorb and scatter light has been utilized by El-Sayed et al to demonstrate the detection and imaging of malignant cells. El-Sayed et al conjugated the anti-body of Epidermal Growth Factor Receptor, which is only expressed by malignant cells onto nanogold. After the absorbtion of the nanogold-anti EGFR conjugate into the cancer cells, the cells were reported to be "shining" in dark field microscopy.

The ability of gold nanoparticles to strongly bind with biological molecules, has been utilized to target cancer tissues by tagging the nanoparticle with a suitable antibody. This antibody-nanogold conjugate are used as vectors for delivering drug molecules or ionizing radiation in the form of radioactive nanogold. Currently the research pursued by Dr. Katti and co-workers in development of hybrid Gold-198/199 nanoparticulates will deliver effective therapeutic response for treating prostate cancer. Higher therapeutic dose is ensured when nanoparticles of the emitting Gold 198/199 are used. The Hybrid Au-198/199 nanoparticulate conjugates are being prepared by conjugation with prostate cancer specific bombesin peptide analogs. These peptides have high affinity toward receptors on prostate, breast and small cell lung cancer cells.

Many cytotoxic cancer therapeutic drugs have a major disadvantage when longer periods of time, is concerned with its acute toxicity. Dr. Katti and his group have recently developed a new class of Au (I) phosphine complexes. Have demonstrated cytotoxicity against human androgen independent prostatic carcinoma (PC-3 cell line), human androgen dependent carcinoma (LNCap. FGC cell line), human colon carcinoma cells (HCT-15 cell lines) and human gastric carcinoma (AGS).

Subsequently antibiotic coated nanogold for sustained release and functionalized nanogold for mammalian cell transfection, have been developed.

Recent reports mention certain unique intrinsic capabilities of gold nanoparticles in X-ray radiotherapy enhancement in mice-bearing EMT-6 mammary carcinomas. Similarly anti-angiogenesis action, was observed when gold nanoparticles interact selectively with heparin-binding glycoproteins and inhibit angiogenesis.

CytImmune Sciences, Inc. (College Park, MD) is partnering with Octo-Plus (Leiden, the Netherlands) to use colloid gold as a means to deliver the anticancer protein, tumor necrosis factor (TNF), known as Aurimune-T. The scientists have used innovative methods to avoid being detected by the immune system by placing linear pieces of PEG in between the TNF molecule.

They also discovered that the toxicity of biomolecules could be drastically reduced when bound to colloidal gold. Once these particles are in the blood stream they get engulfed in water resulting in a "stealth" effect. The particle size of nanogold is 25 nanometers, small enough to pass through the blood vessels of the tumor (around 100nm in diameter) and large enough to pass through blood vessels of healthy organs (5nm in diameter). The Phase I trials have already commenced in late 2003.

THE NANOSCALE MOLECULAR MACHINES

In 1959, Late Nobel Laurete physicist Dr. Feyman, proposed the concept of developing tools to fabricate smaller tools, again to fabricate smaller structures, this would continue till fabrication level is possible at the atomic level.

"Bottom-Up Synthesis" where molecular components are formed by arrangement of special ordered arrangement of carbon and silicon-based molecules. Similar to a methodology of automobile assembly line, the molecular components are assembled into a nanomachine. Drexler proposed the concept of a molecular assembler which could assemble the nanomachines or make copies of themselves. Martel and co-workers have investigated using a group of independently mobile wireless instrumented microrobot manipulators called Nano-Walkers, to collectively form a nanofactory system to be used for positional manufacturing operations.

Nanomachines with the ability to manipulate cellular organelles and deliver therapeutics or conduct surgery at cellular level, are still at the research phase.

Such nanobots would have to be fabricated by assembling its nano-sized components made comprised of. Successful attempts at research stageshave been carried out to control the mechanical parts of the nanobots and to maneuver them in the desired path using forces from magnetic fields.

Engineering innovations in laser technology has opened new horizons in optical nanosurgery. Using femtolasers that behave similarly to a pair of "nano-scissors", perform incision on precise desired locations, leaving adjacent area unharmed. Research in such type of optical nano-scissors range from nanosurgery of focal adhesions in mammalian cells, to dissection of cellular membranes and elimination of intended cell organelles and even to the extent of selectively knocking out genomic regions.

Nano and Micro-sized Systems for Diagnosis, Treatment and Invasive Procedures

In comparison to the intended application of futuristic surgical nanomachines, similar functions can be carried out by devices based on micro/submicron technologies using silicon or engineered polymers. The existence of advanced and low cost semiconductor and microchip manufacturing technologies has provided scientists and researchers to develop micron-sized sensors and actuator systems known as micro/nano electro-mechanical systems (MEMS and NEMS).

Collaborative research endeavors are being initiated to develop a prototype nanoscale assembler, using a NEMS developed by micro-scale scale technologies (Concept of Feyman Nanotechnology). Zyvex Corp. of Richardson, TX has a $25 million, five-year, National Institute of Standards and Technology (NIST) contract to develop prototype micro-scale assemblers using MEMS.

Bio-MEMS

Such systems have been used as a diagnostic tool in cancer therapy, by incorporation of novel-functional or novel-shaped nanomaterials and biomolecular markers, Popularly known as nano/microsensor chips and Bio-chips such as the DNA chip. Nanoscale devices are developed to manipulate biomolecules and also interface with complex biological systems. This makes possible to study the fundamental biological mechanisms that dictate health and disease. This opens a new horizon where nanomedicines can be synthesized based on the cell-molecular machinery and signal transduction mechanisms, artificial cells, targeted molecular drug delivery combined with therapeutic imaging.

Nanowires made out of carbon, silicon and other materials, which have the property of specificity and selectivity are incorporated in microfludic devices. When sample solution particles flow through the microfluidic channel, the nanowire senses, recognizes the molecular signatures of these particles and immediately relays the information, through a connected network of electrodes and electronics. This technique can be used for detection of altered genes. Biomolecular markers loaded onto micron-sized cantilevers, undergo deformation based on the number of target molecules bound to the biomarker. This in turn is calibrated for different concentrations of the target molecule.

BIOSENSORS BASED ON CELLS

Multiple biochemical pathways are performed to translate the molecular code on the oncogene into a malignant tissue. Detection or identification of the key molecules in such pathways is often difficult using engineered molecules or integrating engineered molecules into Silicon Microsystems (Biosensors).

Instead a living cell can be integrated in a microsystem as the primary transduction mechanism. The cells would detect the key bio-chemicals, as they themselves are chemical factories/labs laboratories and can amplify a chemical signal. This can be detected by either monitoring physical parameters (such as electrical activity, structural changes) or chemical parameters (production of "messenger" molecules). Though limitations to incorporate such microsystems would include robustness of the living cells, possible contamination by cell/bacteria in the body and short life cycle of the cells. Still it has demonstrated a considerable good performance for in-vitro studies.

For example: One sensor uses chick myocardial cells to detect the presence of epinephrine, verapamil and tetrodotoxin in the cell environment. Limitations of cell-based sensors include the lifetime and robustness of the cells.

Treatment, Manipulation and Study of Malignant Tissues

Malignant tissues and tumors, such as squamous cell carcinoma are difficult to remove during surgical treatment due to their hardness. Even by using microactuators to surgically interact with such tissues would rather be less effective as are unable to withstand forces on the scale of ~1 mN.

Instead Ultrasonic Piezoelectric actuators attached to the scalpel /surgical cutter, resonate at the tip of the tool at ultrasonic frequencies, to assist in rapidly cutting through tough and hardened malignant tissues. Similarly Kirson and co-workers have developed a vibrating micropipettes (100 Hz and < 1-mm tip diameter) that can completely cut dendrites from single neurons without affecting cell viability.

Micro-strip (micro-millimeter size range) antennas based on the MEMS technology have been developed for hyperthermia applications by Bernhard and co-workers. The small size and novel structuring of the antennas provide enhanced focusing of the RF (Radio-Frequency) /Microwave radiation for effective heat treatment of the tumors.

The incorporation of MEMS/NEMS (novel semiconductor devices) for monitoring and management of neuronal activity. Here Varadan and co-workers have used an implantable MEMS/NEMS-(Electro-active polymer actuators and microsensors attached to the body) based electrodes wirelessly connected to a sensor network for feedback control mechanism. This was for Deep Brain Stimulation for patients suffering from Parkinson's disease, epilepsy etc. When the sensors sense an abnormal motor activity in the patient, the sensors provide necessary control pulses, which are processed to actuate the implanted actuator in order to control the abnormal activity. This technology can be extended towards pain control and management, for patients suffering from chronic pain during cancer therapy sessions. The biggest advantage being that such wirelessly communicated systems can monitor pain condition of patients via internet, cell phones and PDAs. This would assist medical professionals to tackle patient problems in emergency cases with limited medical staff.

The recently developed "smart pill" (26 mm × 36 mm) an ingestible medical device for imaging and studying the gastro-intestinal tract began its clinical testing in late 2005. This technology based on advanced semi-conductor technology can be used for studying GIT malignancies more closely and conveniently than conventional endoscopy.

With the advancement of MEMS, NEMS and nanoelectronics there is room for enhancement of maneuvering, signal/image-processing, image-capturing and wireless signal transmission from the "smart pill". In this case size reduction (beyond optimum size) can be considered by increasing the performance and stability of the device.

On similar lines of the "smart pill", miniaturized millimeter-sized remotely controlled devices known as "nanorobots", can reach out to inaccessible locations in the human body to obtain high resolution images and diagnose cancer/take tissue samples for biopsy.

Currently Prof. Moshe Shoham's Group at Technion Israel is developing a nanorobot for studying the spinal fractures. (Reported in Daily Mail UK 14th November 2006 in a article titled "Robot that swims up your spine to take pictures of fractures" By Roger Dobson). Their group has developed their own version of the "smart pill" known as Pilcam.

While Adriano Cavalcanti and co-workers are using an innovative approach to develop a nanorobot for diagnosis of cancer before metastases. They plan to incorporate a higher gradient of signal intensity of E-cadherin for chemical parameter identification in guiding nanorobots to identify malignant tissues. The nanorobot would use chemical signals and targeted proteins improve treatment intervention time to identify tumor cells. The group has also developed a virtual reality using clinical data coupled with a real time 3-D environment for validation of their model.

In the near future, the multipurpose nano/microrobots would be equipped with nano/micro-sized instruments for minimal and safe invasive treatment and diagnostic procedures. The accessory instruments of imaging and wireless operation would enable us to conduct real time study of administered therapeutics and treatment procedures.

UPCOMING MULTIDISCIPLINARY AND SUPPORTIVE NANOTECHNOLOGIES

When interdisciplinary innovations from basic sciences and applied engineering are included with nanotechnology, it results in development of miniaturized and low cost instruments for cancer treatment and diagnostics.

The best example is of Dr. Otto Zhou and his co-workers from the University of North Carolina Chapel Hill, who are optimizing their new technology of carbon nanotube (CNT) based X-ray machines, which is smaller in size, low in cost and provides clearer images and operates at lower temperatures as compared to metallic filaments in conventional X-ray machines.

In 2000, after filing the first patent on CNT-based X-ray source, Zhou et al co-founded a company, Xintek, to develop and commercialize the technology.

CNT due to small diameters (in nanometers) easily emits electrons when a small voltage is applied, resulting in low temperature requirement for field emission.

Hence the X-ray machine can be operated at room temperatures, so it is free from bulky ventilation and insulation. This permits the X-ray source to last longer than metal filaments, making the instrument smaller in size and portable. The electrical and thermal properties provide advantage of negligible warm up and cool down timing so that the CNT X-ray machine can take multiple images in fast succession such as a high-speed camera for applications such as X-ray imaging of a beating heart. The high-speed imaging has the potential to make breast compression unnecessary in breast mammography. Recently Zhou et al have developed a micro-CT canner using CNT X-ray tubes in-vivo cancer imaging in small animal models. (Endevours Magazine UNC Chapel Hill Fall 2005)

Similarly by engineering CNTs physical and chemical properties, has made CNT become a potential promising candidate for cellular research and cell level therapeutics. They have shown to be engulfed intracellular by endocytosis and functionalized versions of such CNT's have demonstrated photothermal ablation of cancer cells during in-vitro studies.

SUMMARY

Nanotechnology-based cancer therapeutics and diagnostics, over the past decade, has evolved from nano-sized drug particles to functional nanomaterials that are capable of delivering heat, ionizing radiation and chemotherapeutic agents. Currently these are the only nanotechnology innovations that are feasible in terms of improvised treatment and cost-effectiveness. By incorporating multidisciplinary engineering innovations in nanotechnology, an avenue for development of enhanced, miniaturized and low cost diagnostic/ imaging instruments and treatment machines has opened. The future possibility of tackling "pain-the bitter side of cancer therapy", through nanotechnology would be considered one of the biggest breakthroughs.

The investments for research and development and performance trials are considerably large. Hence the sponsoring agencies both private and government should develop innovative management and economic strategies to make these nanotechnology innovations more cost-effective and ease of availability for patients across all economic classes. Similar approach is advised for the upcoming miniaturized technologies (within sub millimeter and sub-micron) from diverse and interdisciplinary engineering sectors of electronics, mechanical and robotics, which can open new horizons in revolutionizing existing methods of cancer study, diagnosis and treatment. Strong initiatives and new evolved policies should be formed by the Health Departments in collaborations with relevant government or private organizations to provide subsidized cancer nanotechnology therapeutics. The subsidy should also be extended to innovations from non-nanotechnology sector, which support and/ or enhance the performance of cancer nanotechnology innovations.

Studies on the clinical and environmental safety aspects should be conducted extensively. Also predictive models must be developed to forecast long-term toxicities and future possible hazards of nanotechnology innovations that are proven clinically and environmentally safe. This would assist relevant environmental and health safety enforcement bodies to counter any possible near or future threats. It is imperative that relevant ethical issues must be discussed and suitable policies be introduced to avoid violation of human and animal safety norms. The cancer nanotechnology innovations that comply with clinical and environmental safety norms, should be recognized by Medical Insurance Schemes. This would enable medical insurance policy holders to avail benefits of new, upcoming and safe cancer nanotechnology innovations.

The future holds lot of promises as nanotechnology has the potential to provide cancer therapy by challenging the barriers of prohibitive costs and undesirable side-effects.

5

Novel Polymeric Anticancer Agents

Conjugates tested clinically so far have incorporated only established chemotherapeutic agents, including doxorubicin, paclitaxel, camptothecins and platinates. Clinical proof of the concept is now paving the way for synthesis of second-generation conjugates containing experimental chemotherapy and novel polymer-based combinations. Recently synthesised conjugates designed for lyso-somotropic delivery contain novel antitumour agents, such as compounds that have failed in early clinical development due to unacceptable toxicity (e.g. ellipticines (Searle et al. 2001) and TNP-470 (Satchi-Fainaro et al. 2004), or interesting novel natural product antitumour agents (e.g. geldanamycin derivatives (Nishiyama et al. 2003), 1,5-diazaanthraquinones (Vicent et al. 2004a) and wortmannin (Varticovski et al. 2001)). In all cases, HPMA copolymers of traditional structure (molecular weight characteristics and a Gly-Phe-Leu Gly linker) have been used as a platform, with the terminal linker dependent on compound chemistry. HPMAcopolymer-TNP470 (Satchi-Fainaro et al. 2004) is the first polymer-based antiangiogenic agent, and it shows considerable promise in vivo.

While many are beginning to explore novel polymer architectures, including dendrimers as carriers of anticancer agents (Malik et al. 1999), the most pressing need is design of new biodegradable polymeric carriers that can be used at relatively high molecular weight to promote greater EPR-mediated targeting and then safely eliminated. Our recent studies have explored dextrin, a natural polymer degraded by amylase (Hreczuk-Hirst et al. 2001), and pendant chain functionalised polyacetals that display pH-dependent degradation after internalisation into the endosomal or lysosomal compartment (Tomlinson et al. 2002, 2003). These polymers can incorporate the drug (e.g. doxorubicin) via pendant linkage or as a component of the polymer main chain (Vicent et al. 2004b). In the context of endocrine-related cancer, we have recently described diethylstilboestrol (DES) conjugate with DES as a component of the polymer backbone. Although this relatively old agent was used as a model compound, a new concept of anticancer drug delivery was established (Vicent et al. 2004b). These polymeric prodrugs incorporate DES into the polymer main chain in such a way that after endocytic internalisation the conjugates undergo pH-dependent degradation (much faster rates of DES release are seen at acidic pH) to liberate principally the bioactive trans-DES form. Polyacetal DES showed enhanced in vitro cyto-toxicity compared to free DES, indicating potential for further evaluation in vivo where EPR-mediated targeting can be exploited to deliver higher tumour DES concentrations selectively.

Two-step anticancer treatments, such as polymer enzyme polymer prodrug therapy (PDEPT), have also been developed with the advantage of a burst of drug release in the tumour interstitium. In this case, a polymer-enzyme conjugate is prepared (PEGylated enzymes are already in routine clinical use that will hydrolyse selectively a polymer drug linker within the tumour interstitium. The concept of PDEPT was exemplified first by an HPMA copolymer cathepsin B-PK1 combination (Satchi et al. 2001), and subsequently a non-mammalian enzyme linker combination HPMA copolymer-ß-lactamase combined with HPMA-copolymer-glycine-glycine-cephalosporin-doxorubicin (Satchi-Fainaro et al. 2003). We have also shown that HPMA copolymer-bound phospholipases can also be used to modulate drug liberation from liposomes (Duncan et al. 2001). This strategy has been called polymer-enzyme liposome therapy (PELT).

POLYMER CONJUGATES: RATIONALE FOR DESIGN

Although many are aware of the emergence of liposomal and antibody-based products, there is still little appreciation of the growing list of polymer therapeutics used as medicines. Commercialisation of polymer-protein conjugates (such as polyethyleneglycol (PEG)-Lasparaginase (Oncaspar) and PEGylated-recombinant methionyl human granulocyte colony stimulating factor (G-CSF) (Neulasta) in the USA (Harris & Chess 2003), coupled with the transfer of the N-(2-hydroxypropyl)methacrylamide (HPMA) copolymer-doxorubicin conjugate (PK1, FCE28068 into clinical trials in Europe in 1994 (Duncan 2003b, 2005a), has been the breakthrough that led to the exponential growth of interest in this field.

The term 'polymer therapeutics' describes several distinct classes of agent, including polymeric drugs, polymer-drug conjugates, polymer-protein conjugates, polymeric micelles to which drug is covalently bound, and the multicomponent polyplexes that are now being developed as non-viral vectors (reviewed in Duncan 2003a).

They are all considered 'new chemical entities' by regulatory authorities, more like therapeutic antibodies and their conjugates than DDS, which simply non-covalently entrap their drug payload. Over the last decade, more than 10 water-soluble polymer-drug conjugates (sometimes best visualised as macromolecular prodrugs) have entered phase I/II clinical trials as i.v. administered anticancer agents. These include six conjugates based on N-(2-hydroxypropyl)methacrylamide (HPMA) copolymers and, more recently, a series of PEG and polyglutamic acid conjugates. The evolution of this field has been reviewed in Duncan (2003a,b, 2005a,b).

The concept of polymer-anticancer conjugates was first proposed in 1975 (Ringsdorf 1975), and the biological rationale for their design (Duncan & Kopecek 1984, Duncan 1992) and current understanding of the mechanism of action is well documented (Duncan 2003b, 2005a). Briefly, these macromolecular prodrugs comprise a minimum of three components: a natural or synthetic, water-soluble polymeric carrier (usually of 10 000-100 000 Da), a biodegradable polymer-drug linkage (often a peptidyl or ester linkage) and a bioactive antitumour agent. Not surprisingly, the first conjugates synthesised in the 1970s and early 1980s incorporated the most important anticancer agents of that era, particularly anthracycline antibiotics (daunorubicin and doxorubicin), alkylating agents (cyclophosphamide and melphalan) and antimetabolites (methotrexate and 5-fluorouracil).

Normally polymer-drug conjugates achieve tumour-specific targeting by the enhanced permeability and retention (EPR) effect (Matsumura & Maeda 1986). Hyperpermeable angiogenic tumour vessels allow preferential extravasation of circulating macromolecules and liposomes, and once in the interstitium they are retained there by lack of intratumoural lymphatic drainage. This leads to significant tumour targeting (>10-100-fold compared to free drug) and levels up to 20% dose/g have been reported for HPMA copolymer-doxorubicin conjugates, depending on tumour size. Both polymer-and tumour-related characteristics govern the extent of EPR-mediated targeting.

Smaller tumours exhibit the highest concentration of polymer-drug. Using HPMA copolymer fractions in the range 10 000-800 000 Da as probes (Seymour et al. 1995, Noguchi et al. 1998), we found that tumour uptake of polymers (usual molecular diameter 5-20 nm) had broad size tolerance and good intratumoural penetration compared with that reported for liposomes and nanoparticles. Conjugates have also been synthesised to contain ligands that might promote receptor-mediated targeting (including antibodies, peptides and saccharides) (reviewed in Duncan 2005a,b). Although this is an attractive possibility, and proof of concept can easily be verified in vitro, so far only one such conjugate has progressed into phase I trial, and this was HPMA copolymer-doxorubicin-galactosamine, which was designed as a treatment for hepatocellular carcinoma or secondary liver disease (PK2, FCE28069 (Seymour et al. 2002).

The growing database of in vitro, in vivo and clinical data allows reappraisal of our current understanding of the mechanism of action of HPMA copolymeranticancer conjugates (Duncan 2005a). The mechanism of action is complex, and it is clear that many factors act in concert to produce the antitumour effect observed in vivo. Drug pharmacokinetics are profoundly changed after polymer conjugation. After i.v. administration, the conjugate is initially retained in the vascular compartment, so that drug t is increased and the levels of free drug detected in plasma are very low (>100-1000 times less than seen for the conjugated drug). Preclinical rodent pharmacokinetic studies and clinical pharmacokinetics correlate well (reviewed in Duncan 2003b, 2005a). The plasma half-life of HPMA copolymer anticancer conjugates is typically 1-6 h, and elimination occurs predominantly via the kidney; over 50% of conjugated drug is excreted within 24 h. Only in the case of the hepatocyte-targeted conjugate PK2 does hepatobiliary elimination play a major role after liver targeting.

This altered biodistribution reduces drug access to potential sites of toxicity, including the heart and bone marrow. This, together with the enhanced elimination of inactive, conjugated drug via the kidney (when the polymer-drug linker is stable), explains the significant reduction in toxicity of anticancer conjugates such as PK1 and PK2 in man (Vasey et al. 1999, Seymour et al. 2002). Gamma camera imaging has shown some evidence to support EPR174-mediated tumour localisation in patients (Vasey et al. 1999). However, when colorectal cancer patients were given HPMA copolymer-camptothecin (MAG-CPT) 24 h before surgical removal of the tumour, the levels of conjugate measured in tumour tissue did not show preferential localisation compared to normal tissue (Sarapa et al. 2003).

Further studies are needed in the clinical setting to clarify the clinical significance of the EPR effect in human tumours of different tissue origin and the extent of targeting at different stages of tumour development (primary, metastatic, postsurgery, etc.). Not least, we need to understand more about the effect of different dosing protocols and combinations with drug and/or radiotherapy on clinically related, EPR-mediated targeting.

Observations made in preclinical and clinical studies underline the need for careful design of the polymer drug linker so that it is stable in transit and degraded at a suitable rate intratumourally (reviewed in Duncan 2003b, 2005a). With HPMA copolymer conjugates, the lysosomally degradable peptidyl linkers (activated by thiol-dependant proteases) have shown the most promise. Hydrolytically labile terminal ester bonds have also been used to prepare conjugates of paclitaxel and camptothecin, and pH-sensitive hydrazone or cis-aconityl linkers are also currently being explored preclinically. A variety of terminal ligands have been used to synthesise HPMA copolymer-platinates with cisplatin-'like' (Gianasi et al. 1999), carboplatin-'like' (Gianasi et al. 2002) and oxaliplatin-'like' structure.

Whichever linking chemistry is used, it is important to note that there is a clear influence of drug loading on conjugate conformation in solution. This in turn governs drug release rate and consequently therapeutic index. High loading with hydrophobic drugs can reduce the rate of prodrug activation, and solution conformation determines rates of both hydrolytic and enzymatic degradation.

Not only does drug conjugation affect whole-body pharmacokinetics, but it also changes fate at the cellular level. While many low-molecular-weight compounds enter tumour cells rapidly (within minutes) by passage across the plasma membrane, polymer conjugates are taken into cells much more slowly by endocytosis (reviewed in Duncan 2005a,b). This frequently makes comparative in vitro screening of activity almost meaningless.

Conjugates containing free drug as a contaminant or that rapidly off-load drug in the tissue culture medium appear most potent. These conjugates, however, are often the least likely to exhibit a good therapeutic index in vivo. Endocytic internalisation of conjugates has been verified with a variety of cell lines, using 125I-labelled probes, HPLC assay of drug, and both epifluorescence and confocal microscopy. This route of cellular entry appears to enable agents to bypass efflux pump-mediated MDR.

There is growing evidence to support an immunostimulatory action of HPMA copolymer anticancer conjugates (reviewed in Duncan 2005a). Rihova has postulated that the early antitumour activity in vivo occurs via cytotoxic or cytostatic action, but that secondary immunostimulatory action of circulating low levels of conjugate supplement this effect (Rihova et al. 2003). This hypothesis is supported by the following evidence:

1. It is observed that pretreatment of animals with immunosuppressive agents (such as doxorubicin and cyclosporine A) accelerates the growth of subsequently implanted tumour, whereas pretreatment with HPMA copolymer-doxorubicin does not.
2. An increase in circulating natural killer (NK) cell numbers and anticancer antibodies is seen in animals treated with conjugate.
3. Increased NK and lymphokine activated killer (LAK) cells have been seen in breast cancer patients treated with HPMA copolymer-Dox-IgG (Rihova et al. 2003).

CLINICAL STATUS OF POLYMER-DRUG CONJUGATES

In 1994, the first synthetic polymer-anticancer conjugate entered clinical trial. This was HPMA copolymer-Gly-Phe-Leu-Gly-doxorubicin (PK1, FCE28068. It has a molecular mass of ~30 000 Da and a doxorubicin content of ~8.5 wt% (Vasey et al. 1999). This peptidyl linker was designed to be hydrolysed by thiol-dependent proteases (particularly cathepsin B) after lysosomotropic delivery.

In phase I trials, PK1 was administered as a short infusion every 3 weeks, and it had a maximum tolerated dose of 320 mg/m2 (doxorubicin equivalent) (Vasey et al. 1999). This is approximately fourfold higher than the normal safe clinical dose of doxorubicin, and a much higher anthracycline dose than can be safely given in liposomal form. The FCE28068dose-limiting toxicities were typical of the anthracyclines, including febrile neutropenia and mucositis. Despite cumulative doses up to 1680 mg/m2 (doxorubicin equivalent), no cardiotoxicity was observed. Antitumour activity was seen in patients considered chemotherapy resistant/refractory (including breast cancer) and at lower doxorubicin doses (80-180 mg/m2). Activity at the lower dose was consistent with EPR-mediated targeting.

Despite a large number of research studies exploring ligand-targeted polymer conjugates (reviewed in Duncan 2005a), PK2 (FCE28069 is still the only targeted conjugate to be tested clinically (Seymour et al. 2002). It was designed to recognise the hepatocyte asialoglyco-protein receptor and has been explored as a treatment for hepatocellular carcinoma. In phase I/II, the maximum tolerated dose of FCE28069 was 160 mg/m^2 (doxorubicin equivalent). Gamma camera imaging confirmed that most of the conjugate localised to liver. The majority of conjugate was present in normal liver (after 24 h, 16.9% dose) with lower accumulations within hepatic tumour (3.2% dose). However, it was estimated that this hepatoma-associated drug was still 12-50 fold higher than could be achieved with administration of free doxorubicin. Antitumour activity was seen in patients with primary hepatocellular carcinoma in this study.

Clinical studies with an HPMA copolymer-paclitaxel conjugate (PNU166945) and HPMA copolymer-camptothecin (MAG-CPT; PNU 166148) were disappointing. In both cases, this was probably due to lack of ester linker stability during transport in the circulation and/or renal elimination. HPMA copolymer-paclitaxel showed toxicity consistent with commonly observed paclitaxel toxicities: flu-like symptoms, mild nausea and vomiting, mild haematological toxicity and neuropathy (Meerum Terwogt et al. 2001). Neurotoxicity grade 2 occurred in two patients at a dose of 140 mg/m^2 (although grade 1 was pre-existing on their entry), and one patient at 196 mg/m2 had grade 3 neuropathy after the fourth cycle.

Although no dose limiting toxicities (DLTs) were reported, dose escalation was discontinued prematurely due to concerns of potential clinical neurotoxicity. In this small patient cohort, antitumour activity was also observed. A paclitaxel-refractory breast cancer patient showed remission of skin metastasis after two courses at 100 mg/m^2 (paclitaxel equivalent). Two other patients had stable disease at a dose of 140 mg/m2. PNU166148 (MAG-CPT) containing Gly-C6-Glycamptothecin showed severe and unpredictable cystitis in phase I clinical trials, and cumulative bladder toxicity was dose limiting. No objective clinical responses were seen; however, one patient with renal cell carcinoma had tumour shrinkage and a colon patient had stable disease (Schoemaker et al. 2002).

HPMA copolymer platinates (Rademaker-Lakhai et al. 2004), polymeric micelles containing doxorubicin and paclitaxel (Nakanishi et al. 2001), and PEG-camptothecin and paclitaxel conjugates (Greenwald et al. 2003) are also undergoing early clinical evaluation.

However, the polymer conjugate most advanced in clinical development is a polyglutamate-paclitaxel conjugate (Li et al. 1998, Auzenne et al. 2002) called Xyotax, which is being developed by Cell Therapeutics (Seattle, WA, USA). An extensive phase II/III evaluation is under way, focusing on non small cell lung cancer (NSCLC) patients being treated with Xyotax as either a single agent (compared with paclitaxel, gemcitabine or vinorelbine) or in combination with carboplatin. Earlier phase I/II studies have reported very interesting activity in NSCLC and also relapsed ovarian cancer. Several phase III clinical trials are currently concluding , and the Gynecologic Oncology Group (GOG) in the USA has recently initiated a phase III clinical trial involving Xyotax in ovarian cancer patients.

POLYMER CONJUGATES CONTAINING ENDOCRINE AND CHEMOTHERAPY COMBINATIONS

The polymeric carrier provides an ideal platform for delivery of a cocktail of drugs simultaneously. We have recently reported the first endocrine-chemotherapy combination in the form of the model compound HPMA-copolymer-aminoglutethimide-doxorubicin (Vicent et al. 2005).

Here it was hypothesised that combination of endocrine therapy and chemotherapy by simultaneous attachment to the same polymer would bring significant advantages.

The combination can be administered as a single dose, leading to the benefits of manufacture of a single conjugate and improved patience compliance. After EPR-mediated targeting, arrival of both pendant drugs within the tumour cells at the same time is guaranteed.

It also provides the opportunity to tailor polymer-drug linkers to impart different rates of drug release for each compound, allowing agents to act synergistically. In in vitro experiments using MCF-7 cells and an aromatase-transfected cell line MCF-7Ca, it was found that conjugates containing both drugs (aminoglutethimide and doxorubicin) showed markedly enhanced cytotoxicity compared to PK1 (the conjugate that has already shown activity in breast cancer patients clinically), while mixtures of polymer conjugates containing only aminoglutethimide or only doxorubicin did not show synergistic benefit. These observations underline the possibility of designing polymer-drug combinations for improved treatment of breast and prostate cancer.

DENDRITIC POLYMERS

Dendritic polymers are materials with a highly branched structure. They combine unique chemical and physical properties. Due to the large number of endgroups-one at every end of a branch-they are highly functional. The high degree of branching prevents crystallization. The materials are soluble in numerous organic solvents. Furthermore, the high degree of branching renders entanglement of the polymers impossible, which results in low melt and solution viscosity.

Over the past decade, perfect dendrimers have received immense interest from academic as well as industrial researchers. However, commercial applications of these perfectly branched materials are scarce, since the tedious multistep synthesis result in inacceptable costs for most applications.

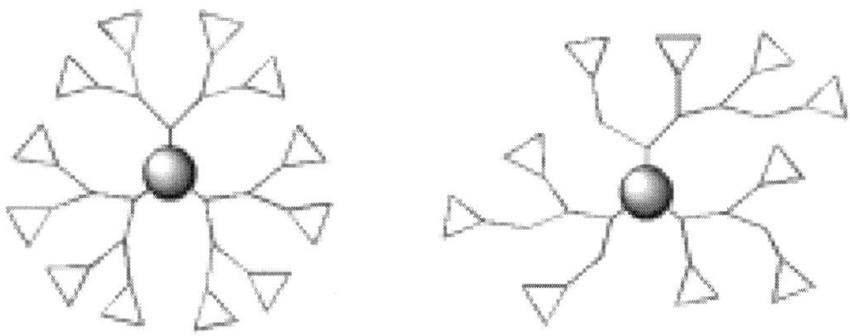

Schematic comparison between a perfect dendrimer and a hyperbranched polymer with a central core (o) and multiple functional endgroups (Δ) in the periphery. The so-called hyperbranched materials also contain a large number of branches. However, they are not perfectly (i.e. absolutely regularly) branched. In this respect their structure can be compared to a tree, which also contains larger and smaller branches. In contrast to dendrimers, hyperbranched polymers can be prepared conveniently in one-step procedures. However, due to extremely broad molecular weight distributions and undesired side reactions, such polymers were regarded as very ill-defined materials. The simultaneous presence of large fractions of low molecular weight compounds and high molecular weight polymers is inacceptable for most applications.

HYPERBRANCHED POLYGLYCEROL

Synthesis Only recently, a synthetic route enabling the preparation of well-defined hyperbranched polyglycerols was discovered in Freiburg. A proprietary process affords polyglycerols with narrow molecular weight distribution ($Mw/Mn < 1.5$) and defined molecular weights in the range of 1.000 to 30.000 g/mol. Currently, the production process is run on a kilogramm scale. There are no basic concerns or prohibitions regarding further scale-up, and the technical realization is in progress

Chemical Properties and Structure: Hyperbranched polyglycerol possesses an inert polyether scaffold. Each branch ends in a hydroxy-function, which renders hyperbranched polyglycerol a highly functional material, e.g., a molecule with a molecular weight of 5000 g/mol possesses 68 hydroxyl end groups. The high functionality in combination with the versatile and well-investigated reactivity of hydroxyl-functions is the basis for a variety of derivatives. Partial esterification with fatty acids yields amphiphilic materials, which behave as nanocapsules. Such nanocapsules can, for example, incorporate polar molecules as guests and solubilize them in an apolar environment.

Selective modification can be achieved utilizing the reactivity of 1,2-diol units, located preferentially at the periphery of the molecule. Complementary to functionalization by reactions of the large number of hydroxy-groups, a single functionality can also be introduced selectively as the 'core' of the molecule. A number of single core functionalities, such as a vinylic group, amines and thiols, have been incorporated.

As alluded to, by using an appropriate protocoll for their synthesis hyperbranched polyglycerols can be prepared with controlled molecular weights. Molecular weights currently available are in the range of 1.000 up to 30.000 g/mol (true molecular weights, determined by various methods). Molecular weight distributions are narrow, that is the apparent polydispersity Mw/Mn is usually below 1.5 (determined by size exclusion chromatography vs. polypropyleneoxide standards). Physical properties. Hyperbranched polyglycerol is a clear, viscous liquid. The glass transition temperature is considerably below room temperature, typically around Tg-25 °C. At room temperature it is highly viscous, the viscosity increasing with molecular weight. By simple heating to slightly elevated temperatures (80°C) it behaves like a free-flowing liquid. Hyperbranched polyglycerol is highly soluble in water and also polar organic solvents, such as methanol. By comparison to linear, non-branched polymers solution-viscosity is considerably lower. Polyglycerols are essentially non-volatile at room temperature.

Biocompatibility is one particularly advantageous feature of aliphatic polyether structures, such as polyglycerol. Thus, an essential prerequisite for applications as a delivery agent for biologically active compounds, cosmetics etc. is provided. In containing hydroxy-endgroups and a polyether-backbone, the hyperbranched polyglycerols resemble the well-known linear polyethylene glycols (PEG, PEO) which are approved for a large variety of medical and biomedical applications.

HYPERBRANCHED POLYETHYLENIMINE

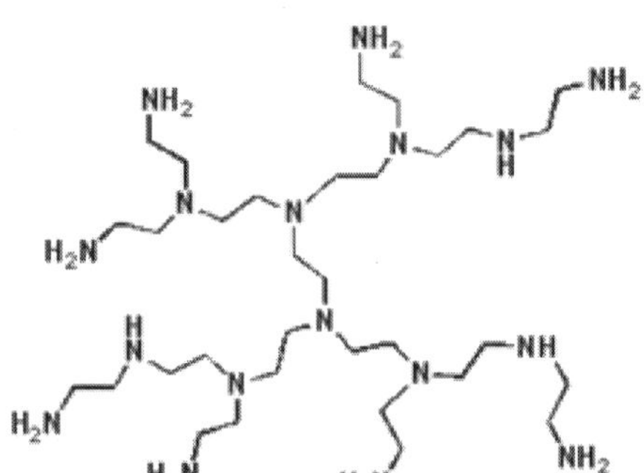

Dendritic polyethylenimine is a highly functional aliphatic polyamine with a globular structure. It has a degree of branching between 65-75% and relatively narrow polydispersities (ca. 1.3 for PEI-5 and ca. 2.5 for PEI-25). It is a transparent colorless viscous liquid with a low intrinsic viscosity in solution.

Targeted Pharmaceutical Nanocarriers

The use of various pharmaceutical nanocarriers has become one of the most important areas of nanomedicine. Ideally, such carriers should be specifically delivered (targeted) to the pathological area to provide the maximum therapeutic efficacy. Among the many potential targets for such nanocarriers, tumors have been most often investigated. This review attempts to summarize currently available information regarding targeted pharmaceutical nanocarriers for cancer therapy and imaging. Certain issues related to some popular pharmaceutical nanocarriers, such as liposomes and polymeric micelles, are addressed, as are different ways to target tumors via specific ligands and via the stimuli sensitivity of the carriers. The importance of intracellular targeting of drug-and DNA-loaded pharmaceutical nanocarriers is specifically discussed, including intracellular delivery with cell-penetrating peptides.

POLYMERIC MICELLES

The present invention provides a colloidal composition consisting of polymeric micelles which may be used to deliver therapeutic agents which have poor water solubility and/or a specific affinity for the hydrophilic shell. The polymeric micelles are characterized by a core shell structure, wherein a hydrophobic core is surrounded by a hydrophilic shell. The hydrophilic shell comprises a hydrophilic polymer or copolymer.

The hydrophilic polymer of the present invention is a polymer or copolymer of poly(N-vinyl-2-pyrrolidone) (PVP).

The hydrophobic moiety constitutes the core of the micelle. The hydrophobic moiety may be chosen from polyesters, such as poly(glycolic acid), poly(lactic acid), poly (D-lactic acid), poly (D,L-lactic acid), lactide/glycolide copolymers, polycaprolactone and derivatives thereof; poly) orthoesters and derivatives thereof; polyanhydrides and derivatives thereof; tyrosine derived pseudo-poly(amino acids) and derivatives thereof; polyphosphazenes and derivatives thereof; poly(alkylacrylate) and derivatives thereof; poly(.beta.-benzyl-L-aspartate) and derivatives thereof and combinations thereof. A preferred hydrophobic moiety is of poly (D,L-lactide (PDLLA). The PDLLA is present at a concentration varying between about 10% and about 50% (w/w).

Formation of Micelles

Micelle formation occurs as a result of two forces. One is an attractive force that leads to the association of molecules, while the other is a repulsive force that prevents unlimited growth of the micelles to a distinct macroscopic phase. Amphiphilic copolymers self-associate when placed in a solvent that is selective for either the hydrophilic or hydrophobic polymer.

The micellization process of amphiphilic copolymers is similar to that for low molecular weight surfactants. At very low concentrations, the polymers exist only as single chains. As the concentration increases to reach a critical value called the critical association concentration ("CAC"), polymer chains start to associate to form micelles in such a way that the hydrophobic part of the copolymer will avoid contact with the aqueous media in which the polymer is diluted. At the CAC, an important quantity of solvent can be found inside the micellar core, and micelles are described as loose aggregates which exhibit larger size than micelles formed at higher concentrations.

At those concentrations, the equilibrium will favor micelle formation, micelles will adopt their low energy state configuration and the remaining solvent will be gradually released from the hydrophobic core resulting in a decrease in micellar size. Amphiphilic copolymers usually exhibit a CAC which is much lower than that of low molecular weight surfactants. For example, the CAC of PEO-PBLA and PNIPA-PSt are between 0.0005-0.002%. Some amphiphilic copolymers, however, exhibit much higher CAC, reaching up to 0.01-10% in the case of poloxamers. Amphiphilic copolymers with high CAC may not be suitable as drug targeting devices since they are unstable in an aqueous environment and are easily dissociated upon dilution.

The micellization of amphiphilic copolymers can result in two different types of micelles depending on whether the hydrophobic chain is randomly bound to the hydrophilic polymer or grafted to one end of the hydrophilic chain. Micelles formed from randomly modified polymers are generally smaller than end-modified polymers. The micellar size is mainly determined by the hydrophobic forces which sequester the hydrophobic chains in the core, and by the excluded volume repulsion between the chains which limits their size. The difference in the balance of these two forces in random and end-modified copolymers may account for their different size.

When terminal hydrophobic groups associate to form micelles, the water clusters immobilized around the hydrophobic segments are excluded from the core and no direct interaction exists between the core and the hydrophilic shell, which remains as mobile linear chains in the micellar structure. Randomly modified polymers, however, associate in such a manner that the hydrophobic and hydrophilic parts of the polymer are entangled together allowing possible contact between the core and the aqueous medium. This is an important issue, since exposed hydrophobic cores may result in secondary aggregation of polymeric micelles. Secondary aggregation has also been proposed as an hypothesis to explain the presence of large particles (>100 nm) in micellar systems of PEO-P(Asp) bearing conjugated doxorubicin (DOX).

Determination of Critical Association Concentration (CAC)

Light scattering is widely used for the determination of the molecular weight and aggregation number of micelles. The onset of micellization can, however, be detected only if the CAC falls within the sensitivity of the scattering method. This is rarely the case for polymers in water. Gel permeation chromatography (GPC) under aqueous conditions can be employed since single chains and micellar fractions of copolymers exhibit different elution volumes. It is also possible to simultaneously determine by GPC the molecular weight of the micelles and their aggregation number. It is important that the integrity of polymeric micelles be maintained during their elution through the size exclusion column. Adsorption of the polymer on the column may also present a problem, especially at concentrations close to the CAC where micelles consist of large loose aggregates.

A preferred method to determine the CAC involves the use of fluorescent probes, among which pyrene is widely used. Pyrene is a condensed aromatic hydrocarbon that is highly hydrophobic and sensitive to the polarity of the surrounding environment. Below the CAC, pyrene is solubilized in water, a medium of high polarity. When micelles are formed, pyrene partitions preferentially toward the hydrophobic domain afforded by the micellar core, and thus experiences a non-polar environment. Consequently, numerous changes such as an increase in the fluorescence intensity, a change in the vibrational fine structure of the emission spectra, and a red shift of the (0,0) band in the excitation spectra are observed. The apparent CAC can be obtained from the plot of the fluorescence of pyrene, the I1/I3 ratio from emission spectra or the I338/I333 ratio from the excitation spectra versus concentration.

A major change in the slope indicates the onset of micellization. The I1/I3 ratio is the intensity ratio between the first and third highest energy emission peaks and is measured at a constant excitation wavelength and variable emission wavelengths corresponding to I1 and I3. The CAC determined with fluorescence techniques needs to be carefully interpreted for two reasons. First, the concentration of pyrene should be kept extremely low (1031 7 M), so that a change in slope can be precisely detected as micellization occurs. Second, a gradual change in the fluorescence spectrum can sometimes be attributed to the presence of hydrophobic impurities or association of the probe with individual polymeric chains or premicellar aggregates. Changes in anisotropy of fluorescent probes have also been associated with the onset of micellization.

Polymeric micelles such as those of the compositions of the invention are characterized by their small size (10-100 nm). Besides being needed for extravasation of the carrier materials, this small size permits the sterilization of the composition to be effected simply by filtration, and minimizes the risks of embolism in capillaries. This is not the situation encountered with larger drug carriers. Micellar size depends on several factors including copolymer molecular weight, relative proportion of hydrophilic and hydrophobic chains and aggregation number. The size of micelles prepared by dialysis can be affected by the organic solvent used to dissolve the polymer.

Micellar diameter and size polydispersity can be obtained directly in water or in an isotonic buffer by dynamic light scattering (DLS). DLS can also provide information on the sphericity of polymeric micelles.

Micellar size can also be estimated by methods such as atomic force microscopy (AFM), transmission electron microscopy (TEM) and scanning electron microscopy (SEM). These methods allow the characterization of the micelle shape and size dispersity. Ultracentrifugation velocity studies are sometimes performed to assess the polydispersity of polymeric micelles.

Incorporation of Therapeutic Agents into Polymeric Micelles

Loading of a therapeutic agent into the micelles can be realized according to techniques well known to one skilled in the art. For example, loading may be effected by dissolution of the compound in a solution containing preformed micelles, by the oil-in-water procedure or the dialysis method.

Therapeutic agents which may be used are any compounds, including the ones listed below, which can be entrapped, in a stable manner, in polymeric micelles and administered at a therapeutically effective dose. Preferably, the therapeutic agents used in accordance with the invention are hydrophobic in order to be efficiently loaded into the micelles.

However it may be possible to form stable complexes between ionic micelles and oppositely charged hydrophilic compounds such as antisense oligonucleotides. Suitable drugs include antitumor compounds such as phthalocyanines (e.g. aluminum chloride phthalocyanine), anthracyclines (e.g.

doxorubicin (DOX)), poorly soluble antimetabolites (e.g. methotrexate, mitomycin, 5-fluorouracil) and alkylating agents (e.g. carmustine). Micelles may also contain taxanes such as paclitaxel.

Additional drugs which can be contained in micelles are conventional hydrophobic antibiotics and antifungal agents such as amphotericin B, poorly water soluble immunomodulators such as cyclosporin, poorly water soluble antiviral drugs such as HIV protease inhibitors and poorly water-soluble steroidal (e.g. dexamethasone), non-steroidal (e.g. indomethacin) anti-inflammatory drugs and genome fragments.

Further, drugs can be incorporated into the polymeric micelle compositions of the invention by means of chemical conjugation or by physical entrapment through dialysis, emulsification techniques, simple equilibration of the drug and micelles in an aqueous medium or solubilization of a drug/polymer solid dispersion in water.

Hydrophilic compounds such as proteins may also be incorporated in the polymeric micelle compositions of the invention. The incorporation of such hydrophilic species may, however, require the chemical hydrophobization of the molecule or a particular affinity for the hydrophilic shell. Polyionic compounds can be incorporated through the formation of polyionic complex micelles.

Physical entrapment of drugs is generally carried out by a dialysis or oil-in-water emulsion procedure. The dialysis method consists in bringing the drug and copolymer from a solvent in which they are both soluble, such as ethanol or N,N-dimethylformamide, to a solvent that is selective only for the hydrophilic part of the polymer, such as water. As the good solvent is replaced by the selective one, the hydrophobic portion of the polymer associates to form the micellar core incorporating the insoluble drug during the process. Complete removal of the organic solvent may be brought about by extending the dialysis over several days. In the oil-in-water emulsion method, a solution of the drug in a water-insoluble volatile solvent, such as chloroform, is added to an aqueous solution of the copolymer to form an oil-in-water emulsion. The micelle-drug conjugate is formed as the solvent evaporates. The main advantage of the dialysis procedure over the latter method is that the use of potentially toxic solvents such as chlorinated solvents can be avoided.

The drug loading procedure may affect the distribution of a drug within the micelle. For example, Cao et al. (Macromolecules 24 (1991) 6300-6305), showed that pyrene incorporated in micelles as they were forming was not protected from the aqueous environment as well as pyrene incorporated after micelles were formed, although the first method yielded a drug loading three times higher than the second method.

Entrapment efficiency of the polymeric micelles of the invention depends on the initial amount of drug added. Exceeding the maximum loading capacity results in precipitation of the therapeutic agent, and consequently, lower yield. Further, efficiency of loading of the therapeutic agent depends on the aggregation number of copolymer. Micelles showing a higher aggregation number allow a greater amount of drug to be solubilized in their inner core. Multifunctional polymeric micelles with folate-mediated cancer cell targeting and pH-triggered drug releasing properties for active intracellular drug delivery

A new type of multifunctional polymeric micelle drug carrier for active intracellular drug delivery was prepared and characterized in this study. The micelle is a nano-supramolecular assembly with a spherical core-shell structure, and its surface and core were modified with piloting molecules for cancer cells and pH-sensitive drug binding linkers for controlled drug release, respectively. In order to prepare such micelles, self-assembling amphiphilic block copolymers, folate-poly(ethylene glycol)-poly(aspartate hydrazone adriamycin) [Fol-PEG-P(Asp-Hyd-ADR)], were specially designed and synthesized by installing a molecular promoter to enhance intracellular transport, folate (Fol), at the end of the shell-forming PEG chain and conjugating the anticancer drug, adriamycin (ADR), to the side chain of the core-forming PAsp segment through an acid-sensitive hydrazone bond.

Because folate-binding proteins (FBP) are selectively overexpressed on the cancer cell membranes, the folate-bound micelles (FMA) can be guided to the cancer cells in the body, and after the micelles enter the cells, hydrazone bonds are cleaved by the intracellular acidic environment (pH 5-6) so that the drug release profile of the micelles is controlled pH-dependently. In this regard, FBP-binding selectivity of the prepared FMA was evaluated by surface plasmon resonance (SPR) measurements.

The tetrazolium dye method (MTT assay) using human pharyngeal cancer cells (KB cell) revealed that FMA significantly improved cell growth inhibitory activity in spite of a short exposure time due to the selective and strong interaction between folate molecules and their receptors. Subsequent flow cytometric analysis showed that cellular uptake of FMA significantly increased. Consequently, these findings would provide one of the most effective approaches for cancer treatment using intracellular environment-targeting supramolecular drug carriers.

Biologically active materials for cancer chemotherapy are usually selected using cell biology and pharmacology, which provide a rationale for understanding the Absorption, Distribution, Metabolism and Excretion (ADME) of exogenous molecules in the body. A number of studies have claimed that polymer science and supramolecular chemistry can offer the most adequate and suitable means for designing functional nano-bio devices. For these reasons, growing interest is currently focused on the creation of functional polymeric nano-carriers that regulate ADME of drugs at the boundary between biochemistry and nano-technology.

Among such carriers, spherical supramolecular nano-assemblies from amphiphilic block copolymers, called polymeric micelles, have attracted considerable attention in the field of drug delivery systems due to their unique characteristics such as high water-solubility, high drug loading capacity and low toxicity, which are induced by the prolonged circulation in the blood and enhanced accumulation in tumor tissue. In particular, the intracellular environment-sensitive polymeric micelle, that can release the loaded drug, adriamycin (ADR), through sensing pH decreases in the acidic endocytic compartments such as endosomes (pH 5-6) and lysosomes (pH 4-5), has recently been reported to minimize non-specific systemic spread of toxic drugs while maximizing tumor-directed drug delivery efficiency. Indeed, animal studies have elucidated that this type of micelle significantly improves the bioavailability of existing drugs by controlling the drug release profile, inducing high antitumor activity with extremely low drug toxicity and avoiding clearance by the host defense system and uptake by normal tissue. Nevertheless, cell growth inhibitory activity still needs to be improved because the effective dose for cancer treatment using these micelles was relatively high, 4-fold compared with free drugs. However, in vitro activity of most polymer-drug conjugates is known to decrease as their biological behavior, that is involved with cellular uptake by an endocytotic pathway and relatively slow drug release, often works to the disadvantage of exerting drug efficacy compared to free drugs that rapidly move into the cell interior.

Consequently, it is expected that if the macromolecular drug carriers were actively transported inside the cells, the bioavailability of the carriers should increase more than the drug carrier system that simply exploits passive drug delivery. In order to achieve both these goals, the micelles are also required to selectively and strongly interact with targeted cells so that intracellular transport can be controllable. On the basis of this background, we have developed a new type of multifunctional polymeric micelle drug carrier system that will actively enhance its capability to deal with intracellular drug delivery to the targeted cancer cells. In the case of carriers for targeting cancer cells, the fundamental problems such as intracellular transport and the release of incorporated materials are often encountered during the materials' intracellular movement.

These problems are particularly crucial to the carriers in terms of the delivery of materials that should become pharmaceutically effective after entering cells.

To satisfy the former requirement, the micelles we present in this study are equipped with folate-ligands, which are non-immunogenic and stable during transportation in vivo without denaturation. For the latter requirement, the pH-sensitivity that enables selective drug release in intracellular acidic compartments, endosomes (pH 5-6), is used. Folate is a vitamin with low molecular weight (MW = 441.4) and behaves as a ligand because it has high affinity for its receptors (Kd < 1 nM), folate-binding proteins (FBP), that are selectively overexpressed on the surface of cancer cells.

Therefore, its conjugates with an appropriate design can be directed to the cancer cells in the body and internalized in the target cells via receptor-mediated endocytosis. In the meantime, there is notable intracellular behavior of the folate-bound materials after ligand-mediated endocytosis, which distinguishes the folate ligand from other types of ligands such as antibodies, hormones and peptides.

In contrast to the fact that most ligands are internalized and transported to the lysosomes, folate-conjugates remain in recycling endosomes (pH 5-6) or escape into the cytoplasm, and such a characteristic plays a crucial role in accelerating intracellular uptake of the materials by the cell, avoiding the possible effects of lysosomal enzyme action. Therefore, the experimental results discussed in this study will present clear information about the effects of folate ligands on biological activity of the intracellular drug delivery when using the supramolecular drug carriers that are selectively activated in the cell.

The Outcome

Design of the micelles and synthesis of their constituent bifunctional block copolymers.

To prepare the folate-bound micelles, self-assembling amphiphilic block copolymers, folate-poly(ethylene glycol)-block-poly(aspartate hydrazone adriamycin) [Fol-PEG-p(Asp-Hyd-ADR)], were designed and synthesized by developing a new and optimized synthetic protocol of both folate and poly(ethylene glycol) (PEG) to introduce functional groups for conjugation. In general, two methods can be used to conjugate folate onto the surface of the polymeric micelles:

(i) preparation of a surface-activated micelle followed by the conjugation of folate molecules by mixing them in the solution, and

(ii) conjugation of folate molecules onto the constituent block copolymers followed by the preparation of the micelles with folate-bound block copolymers.

The former may be a simple method to prepare the surface-modified micelles. However, it is unlikely to ensure high loading contents of folate molecules because the reaction rate is usually low and a cumbersome process of removing unreacted folate molecules is inevitably required. Moreover, the presence of unreacted ligand molecules, free folate, may hamper the binding between folate-bound micelles and folate-binding proteins (FBP) through competitive interaction. In contrast, the latter method, which was adopted in this study, requires a somewhat complex synthetic route involving the protection of functional groups to prevent side reactions, but has several advantages including quantitative reactions and characterization of the products.

An impediment to the preparation of folate-conjugates, isomerization between inactive-conjugates and active-conjugates, can be overcome, and this is quite crucial when preparing folate-conjugates. It has been reported that isomerization of folate-conjugated derivatives frequently occurs, in the case of DCC-coupling for instance, and affects the FBP-binding selectivity of folic acid. Therefore, the present synthetic route is probably one of the the best ways to conjugate folic acid as well as anticancer drugs with PEG at its-position to maintain FBP-binding activity and hydrazide groups at the drug-binding moiety of the side chain, respectively.

SYNTHESIS OF BLOCK COPOLYMERS AND PREPARATION OF THE FOLATE-BOUND MICELLES

As described above, the micelles were prepared after the synthesis of folate-polymer conjugates to maintain FBP-binding activity. This is achieved by the design of an end-group functionalized folate and PEG.

Treatment of folic acid 1 with an excess amount of trifluoroacetic anhydride in THF produces N_2,10-bis (trifluoroacetyl)-pyrofolic acid 2.21 By adding water, the compound affords N10-(trifluoroacetyl)-pyrofolic acid and can be further transformed to pyrofolic acid via deacylation with K_2CO_3. However, both N10-(trifluoroacetyl)-pyrofolic acid and pyrofolic acid are generally known as isomers, and the two imide carbonyl groups (-carbonyl and pteroic carbonyl) of pyrofolic acid derivatives, N10-(trifluoroacetyl)-pyrofolic acid and pyrofolic acid, can react with nucleophiles. For these reasons, the products were purified to confirm the absence of pteroic acid derivatives by using a preparative HPLC and TLC, and pure folate-hydrazide-BOC (Fol-Hyd-BOC) was successfully collected.

From the GPC analysis, the weight-average molecular weight (Mw) and the molecular weight distribution (Mw/Mn) of-4-(diethoxymethyl)benzyl--amine-poly(ethylene glycol) [aceBz-PEG-NH_2**5**] were determined to be 10 159 and 1.02, respectively. The molecular weight was in accordance with the estimated value calculated from the ratio between monomers and initiators and its distribution was extremely narrow. These results indicate that the polymerization of EO proceeds without any side reactions by using potassium 4-(diethoxymethyl) benzylalkoxide (PDA) as an initiator. The end-group was then checked by ^{1}H-NMR, comparing the peaks of PEG and 4-(diethoxymethyl) benzyl alcohol. The molecular weight was determined to be from the peak intensity ratio of PEG (-OCH_2CH_2-) and benzylacetal [($CH_3CH_2O)_2$CH-], which is in a good agreement with the Mw determined by GPC. The ^{1}H-NMR peak of α-4-(diethoxymethyl)benzyl-poly (ethylene glycol)-poly(β-benzyl-L-aspartate) [aceBz-PEG-PBLA 7] synthesized via ring-opening polymerization of β-benzyl L-aspartate-N-carboxy-anhydride (BLA-NCA) by using 5 as a macromolecular initiator.

In the case of folate-poly(ethylene glycol)-poly(-benzyl-L-aspartate) [Fol-PEG-PBLA 9], the molecular weight and its distribution were 22.673 and 1.142 respectively which were determined by GPC equipped with a UV-VIS detector (360 nm) to confirm the conjugation between folate and PEG. ^{1}H-NMR also supported that the conjugation of folate to PEG was successfully carried out because a peak of aldehyde groups of unreacted PEG was not observed after the reaction. The anticancer drug, adriamycin (ADR), was introduced to Fol-PEG-PBLA block copolymers through an acid-sensitive hydrazone bond, and drug-loading contents and pH-sensitive drug release profiles of the folate-bound pH-sensitive micelle with ADR (FMA) were calculated by reversed phase liquid chromatography referring to a method reported elsewhere.

The compositions of 11 were 12-32-21, denoting that the polymer backbones consist of PEG with the molecular weight of 12 000 g mol-1 for the shell-forming segment, PBLA with 32 repeating units for the core-forming segment, and 21 hydrazide groups that are substituted for benzyl groups of PBLA for drug-binding. 11 formed spherical micelles with 63.4 nm diameters in aqueous solutions, which was confirmed by DLS. In the meantime, the folate-unbound pH-sensitive micelle with ADR (MA) was prepared from α-methoxy-poly(ethylene glycol)-poly(aspartate hydrazone adriamycin) [PEG-p(Asp-Hyd-ADR)] as control.

The compositions of its constituent block copolymer PEG-p(Asp-Hyd-ADR) was 12-37-28, denoting that the polymer backbones consisted of PEG with molecular weight of 12 000 g mol^{-1}, PBLA with 37 repeating units, and 28 hydrazide groups substituted for benzyl groups of PBLA for drug-binding. The number of hydrazide groups for drug-binding was optimized by considering stability and the drug release profile of the micelles. Prepared MA had 65 nm diameters, which were also determined by DLS. The size distribution of the micelles, expressed as polydispersity index (μ/Γ^2), was 0.155 and 0.168 for MA and FMA, respectively.

FBP-binding Selectivity of the Micelles

The FBP-binding effect of FMA was evaluated by surface plasmon resonance (SPR) measurements. For the experiments, FBP was immobilized onto a dextran-coated gold sensor chip, which was freshly prepared for each sample injection. The analysis showed that FMA not only effectively recognized but also strongly bound to the FBP. Interestingly, once it binds, even though excess amounts of free folic acid (500 μg ml^{-1}) were added, FMA was not displaced or detached. On the other hand, when both FMA and free folic acid were injected at the same time, the FBP-binding effect of FMA obviously decreased. These results can be explained by the fact that FMA can bind FBP with a strong multivalent form, and binding sites are saturated and blocked in the presence of free folate molecules. Such characteristic behavior was not shown in the case of MA used as control. Therefore, it is clearly revealed that FMA exhibits selective FBP-binding behavior, and the concept described in this research would be an effective approach for designing environment-sensitive polymeric micelle drug carriers for specific recognition of cancer cells in the body.

BIODEGRADABLE POLYMERIC NANOPARTICLES

Throughout various fields of science and technology, a push towards the use of nano-scale technology is well underway. Nanotechnology has the potential to produce low-cost, self-replicating systems that could revolutionize the scientific landscape. One area where nano-scale work is already well underway is within the field of drug delivery. In drug delivery, nanoparticles are fabricated in order to entrap and deliver specific pharmaceutical agents to various locations within the body. Traditional drug delivery methods include oral and intravenous routes of administration. These methods are still the most widely used today, yet each has its disadvantages. Oral delivery via tablets or capsules is largely inefficient due to exposure of the pharmaceutical agent to the metabolic processes of the body.

Therefore, a larger than necessary dose is often required and the maximum effectiveness of the drug is limited. Traditional intravenous (IV) administration is much more problematic. Specificity for IV injectable drugs is often low, necessitating large amounts of a drug be injected into a patient, creating a high concentration of the drug in the blood stream that could potentially lead to toxic side effects. Nanoparticle drug delivery, utilizing degradable and absorbable polymers, provides a more efficient, less risky solution to many drug delivery challenges. Nanoparticles are generally defined as particles between 10 nanometers (nm) and 1000 nm in size, and can be either spherical or vesicular.

The advantages of using polymeric nanoparticles (PNPs) in drug delivery are many, the most important being that they generally increase the stability of any volatile pharmaceutical agents and that they are easily and cheaply fabricated in large quantities by a multitude of methods. Additionally, the use of absorbable or degradable polymers, such as polyesters, provides a high degree of biocompatibility for PNP delivery systems. This is an essential feature for such potential applications as tissue engineering, which will be briefly discussed later. Furthermore, the use of PNPs allows for design of individual delivery systems for highly specific applications. Among the adaptations that can be made are surface modifications of the polymer, use of different fabrication methods, selection of a variety of pre-existing polymers or copolymers, and formulation of novel polymeric materials. This last possibility is especially exciting, as it may be possible in the future to design specific PNP delivery systems for individuals.

Polymeric nanoparticles have the potential to completely transform drug delivery technology. PNPs represent a significant improvement over traditional oral and intravenous methods of administration in terms of efficiency and effectiveness. Also, PNPs can have engineered specificity, allowing them to deliver a higher concentration of pharmaceutical agent to a desired location.

This feature makes PNPs ideal candidates for cancer therapy, delivery of vaccines, and delivery of targeted antibiotics. Moreover, PNPs can be easily incorporated into other activities related to drug delivery, such as tissue engineering, and into drug delivery for species other than humans. Polymeric nanoparticles are the future of drug delivery technology and represent the best way to increase specificity in pharmaceutical therapy, a key to defeating cancer and other heretofore incurable diseases.

Modulation of Intracellular Ceramide Using Polymeric Nanoparticles

Although multidrug resistance (MDR) is known to develop through a variety of molecular mechanisms within the tumor cell, many tend to converge toward the alteration of apoptotic signaling. The enzyme glucosylceramide synthase (GCS), responsible for bioactivation of the proapoptotic mediator ceramide to a nonfunctional moiety glucosylceramide, is overexpressed in many MDR tumor types and has been implicated in cell survival in the presence of chemotherapy. The purpose of this study was to investigate the therapeutic strategy of coadministering ceramide with paclitaxel, a commonly used chemotherapeutic agent, in an attempt to restore apoptotic signaling and overcome MDR in the human ovarian cancer cell line SKOV3.

Poly (ethylene oxide)-modified poly(epsilon-caprolactone) (PEO-PCL) nanoparticles were used to encapsulate and deliver the therapeutic agents for enhanced efficacy. Results show that indeed the cotherapy eradicates the complete population of MDR cancer cells when they are treated at their IC50 dose of paclitaxel. More interestingly, when the cotherapy was combined with the properties of nanoparticle drug delivery, the MDR cells can be resensitized to a dose of paclitaxel near the IC50 of non-MDR (drug sensitive) cells, indicating a 100-fold increase in chemosensitization via this approach. Molecular analysis of activity verified the hypothesis that the efficacy of this therapeutic approach is indeed due to a restoration in apoptotic signaling, although the beneficial properties of PEO-PCL nanoparticle delivery seemed to enhance the therapeutic success even further, showing the promising potential for the clinical use of this therapeutic strategy to overcome MDR.

Development of a Polymeric Nanoparticle Formulation

Nanotechnology is a very useful tool in the design of drug delivery systems to combat many diseases, where these nano-platforms can aide in target specific localization, controlled release, and multifunctionalization of the therapy.

The use of nanoparticles, colloidal carriers of submicronic (1 m) size is particularly of use in the delivery of therapeutics to tumors. Resulting from the rapid growth of a tumor mass, many tumors present with fenestrated vasculature and poor lymphatic drainage, resulting in an enhanced permeability and retention (EPR) effect. Long circulating nanoparticles can extravasate through these fenestrations to accumulate, and deposit their drug load, specifically at the tumor site.

A great challenge to cancer therapy is the development of cross-resistance to a multitude of chemotherapeutic agents, termed multidrug resistance (MDR). It is believed that the development of MDR in a small subset of cancer cells is the reason for tumor survival despite invasive chemotherapy, a phenomenon that is particularly taxing in the treatment of breast and ovarian cancer, where MDR develops in half of the clinical cases.

Although MDR is known to arise through alterations of several cellular processes in the cancer cell, recent research suggests the importance of alterations in apoptotic (programmed cell death) signaling, rendering the MDR cell impervious to cell death resulting from chemotherapy. This project is aimed at overcoming MDR through a therapeutic strategy that uses polymeric nanoparticles to carry and co-administer an MDR modulator, involved in mending the alterations in apoptotic signaling, with a classical chemotherapeutic to re-sensitize MDR cancers to chemotherapy.

AN EXPLANATION

Objective: The development of multidrug resistance (MDR) in many tumor types is a major barrier to successful anti-cancer therapy. One of the mechanisms that leads to such chemoresistance is inhibition of apoptotic signaling in MDR cancer cells through glycosylation of the apoptotic mediator ceramide. The purpose of this study was to investigate whether MDR could be reverted by co-administering exogenous C6-ceramide with a chemotherapeutic (paclitaxel), co-encapsulated in polymeric nanoparticles to produce a multifunctional anticancer therapy.

Experimental Methods: The experimental approach involved testing efficacy of the therapeutic strategy by quantifiying % cell death of drug sensitive vs. multidrug resistant cancer cells in response to the nanoparticle treatment compared to conventional treatments. Next, apoptotic activity in response to paclitaxel/ceramide co-therapy was quantified using a commercially available apoptosis assay. Lastly, intracellular nanoparticle accumulation and localization was observed by fluorescent microscopy.

Results: Results indicate that nanoparticle delivery of the co-therapy reduces chemoresistance of the MDR cells to paclitaxel 100-fold, to produce a chemosensitivity profile in the MDR cells that is similar to their drug-sensitive counterpart cell-line. Co-therapy of ceramide with paclitaxel appeared to increase apoptotic activity 2 fold in the MDR cells, suggesting that delivery of exogenous ceramide reinstates the apoptotic signal to resensitize MDR cells to chemotherapy.

Conclusions: Altogether, co-administering paclitaxel with ceramide, delivered in polymeric nanoparticles appears to greatly re-sensitize drug resistant ovarian tumor cells to chemotherapy. The results demonstrate the great potential for clinical use of this therapeutic strategy to overcome MDR.

Rapid Transport of Large Polymeric Nanoparticles in Fresh Undiluted Human Mucus

Nanoparticles larger than the reported mesh-pore size range (10-200 nm) in mucus have been thought to be much too large to undergo rapid diffusional transport through mucus barriers. However, large nanoparticles are preferred for higher drug encapsulation efficiency and the ability to provide sustained delivery of a wider array of drugs. We used high-speed multiple-particle tracking to quantify transport rates of individual polymeric particles of various sizes and surface chemistries in samples of fresh human cervicovaginal mucus. Both the mucin concentration and viscoelastic properties of these cervicovaginal samples are similar to those in many other human mucus secretions.

Unexpectedly, we found that large nanoparticles, 500 and 200 nm in diameter, if coated with polyethylene glycol, diffused through mucus with an effective diffusion coefficient (Deff) only 4-and 6-fold lower than that for the same particles in water (at time scale = 1 s). In contrast, for smaller but otherwise identical 100-nm coated particles, Deff was 200-fold lower in mucus than in water. For uncoated particles 100-500 nm in diameter, Deff was 2,400- to 40,000-fold lower in mucus than in water. Much larger fractions of the 100-nm particles were immobilized or otherwise hindered by mucus than the large 200-to 500-nm particles. Thus, in contrast to the prevailing belief, these results demonstrate that large nanoparticles, if properly coated, can rapidly penetrate physiological human mucus, and they offer the prospect that large nanoparticles can be used for mucosal drug delivery.

Treatments for cervicovaginal (CV) tract diseases, often based on drugs delivered to the systemic circulation by pills or injections, typically suffer from low efficacy. For example, systemic chemotherapy is typically the last or strictly concurrent option, after surgery and radiotherapy, for treatment of cervical cancer. In addition, systemic medications can lead to significant adverse side effects when high drug concentrations in the circulation are required to elicit a therapeutic response in the CV tract. To reduce side effects and achieve localized therapy, recent efforts have increasingly emphasized topical drug delivery methods, such as creams, hydrogels, and inserted devices, to deliver therapeutics to the apical side of the cervix epithelium. Apical drug delivery may also be extended to protection against sexual transmission of infections, because neutralizing antibodies and microbicides must act at mucosal surfaces to block the entry of pathogens.

Nanoparticle systems possess desirable features for treatment, including:

(i) sustained and controlled release of drugs locally,

(ii) potential to cross the mucosal barrier due to the nanometric size,

(iii) rapid intracellular trafficking to the perinuclear region of underlying cells, and

(iv) protection of cargo therapeutics from degradation and removal in the mucus.

However, therapeutic and/or diagnostic particles must overcome the mucosal barrier lining the CV tract to reach underlying cells and avoid clearance. Mucins, highly glycosylated large proteins (MDa) secreted by epithelial cells, represent the principal component of the entangled viscoelastic gel that protects the underlying epithelia from entry of pathogens and toxins. Other mucus constituents, such as lipids, salts, macromolecules, cellular debris, and water, work together with mucins to form a nanoscopically heterogeneous environment for nanoparticle transport, where the shear-dependent bulk viscosity is typically 100-10,000 times more viscous than water.

Small viruses up to 55 nm have been shown to diffuse in CV mucus as rapidly as in water; however, a larger virus, 180-nm herpes simplex virus, was slowed 100-to 1,000-fold by CV mucus compared with water, suggesting that the mucus mesh spacing is 20-200 nm. It was also previously reported that polystyrene particles (59-1,000 nm) adhered tightly to cervical mucus, rendering them completely immobile. These observations have suggested that the transport of synthetic polymer nanoparticles, especially those larger than 59 nm, was unlikely to occur efficiently enough to allow access of sustained release particles to underlying epithelium in human mucus-covered tissues.

To investigate and potentially improve the transport of nanoparticles across the CV mucus barrier, we studied the quantitative transport rates of hundreds of individual nanoparticles of various sizes and surface chemistries in human CV secretions. Undiluted mucus at physiologically relevant conditions was obtained by a recently described procedure that uses a menstrual-collection device. Surprisingly, we report that nanoparticles larger than the previously reported CV mucus mesh spacing are capable of rapid transport in CV mucus if they are coated with the mucoresistant polymer, low-molecular-weight polyethylene glycol.

THE RESULTS

Real-Time Transport of COOH-Modified Nanoparticles. We first sought to determine the effect of particle size on transport rates in CV mucus obtained from human volunteers. The hydrodynamic diameters of the particles suspended in water, characterized by dynamic light scattering. The addition of uncoated particle at relatively high concentration (2% particles by weight) to CV mucus caused collapse of the mucus fibers into bundles that trapped the particles and prevented their transport (data not shown). However, low concentration of particles (0.008% particles by weight) did not cause bundling and allowed particle movement [supporting information (SI). Surprisingly, 200-and 500-nm COOH-modified particles (COOH-PS) displayed higher transport rates, as measured by geometric ensemble mean-squared displacements (<MSD>), than otherwise similar 100-nm particles. At a time scale of 1 s, 100-nm COOH-PS particles were 9-and 2-fold slower than 200- and 500-nm COOH-PS particles, respectively. The ensemble-average effective diffusivity (<Deff>) of COOH-PS particles decreases at short time scales, as expected in mucus.

By fitting particle MSD vs. time scale to the equation MSD = 4Do, where Do is the diffusion coefficient independent of time scale, one can obtain an average value for that provides insight into the extent of impediment to particle motion (= 1 for pure unobstructed Brownian diffusion, such as particles in water). Average values were 0.16, 0.36, and 0.43 for 100-, 200-, and 500-nm COOH-PS particles, respectively. Overall, the ensemble-average Deff of 100- , 200-, and 500-nm COOH-PS particles in mucus (at = 1 s) were reduced by 44,000-, 590-, and 4,600-fold compared with the same particles in water.

To begin to understand the mechanistic reasons for the unexpectedly low mobility of 100-nm COOH-PS particles (compared with 200 and 500 nm) across all time scales, we sorted particles based on their calculated Deff (at = 1 s) into 10 groups. Although the fastest 10% of 100-nm COOH-PS particles had approximately similar mean Deff as compared with 200-and 500-nm COOH-PS particles, the mean Deff values for 200-and 500-nm COOH-PS particles were greater than for 100-nm COOH-PS particles for all other subgroups (i.e., the slowest 90% of particles), which accounts for the slower ensemble mobility of 100-nm COOH-PS particles. The Deff of individual particles of all sizes spanned a wide range, with the fastest and slowest particles within each particle size differing by at least 4 orders of magnitude. The considerable heterogeneity in Deff within each group of particles suggested that different mechanisms of particle transport exist. This hypothesis is supported by visual observations of both immobile and rapidly moving particles in the same movie.

Real-Time Transport of PEG-Modified Nanoparticles. PEG, a hydrophilic and uncharged polymer, was covalently attached to the surface of 100-, 200-, and 500-nm particles in an attempt to reduce particle interactions with CV mucus. The extent of PEG attachment was comparable for all particles, as shown by their near-neutral surface charges and similar efficiencies in resisting adsorption of fluorescently labeled avidin. Pegylation greatly increased particle transport rates, as is evident by the 20-, 400-and 1,100-fold higher ensemble MSDs (= 1 s) of 100-, 200-, and 500-nm PEGylated particles (PEG-PS) compared with corresponding COOH-PS particles of the same size. The <Deff> (= 1 s) for 100-, 200-, and 500-nm PEG-PS were reduced by only 2,000-, 6-, and 4-fold compared with that of the expected values for their diffusion in water.

The ensemble Deffs of PEG-PS of all three sizes still decreased with increasing time scale, but only 100-nm PEG-PS experienced extensive obstruction to transport (= 0.31, 0.81, and 0.89 for 100-, 200-, and 500-nm PEG-PS, respectively). PEGylation not only reduced impediment for larger PEG-PS (200 and 500 nm) but also increased the homogeneity of transport compared with similar-sized COOH-PS particles.

Analysis of Transport Mechanisms. For all sizes studied, a large fraction of COOH-PS particles appeared to be immobilized by adhering extensively to CV mucus, resulting in an MSD below the resolution of the microscope. A significant percentage of the remaining COOH-PS particles underwent hindered diffusive motions or transport that is restricted by obstacles in the fluid microenvironment. Consequently, only a small fraction of COOH-PS particles exhibited Brownian or near-Brownian trajectories, whereas such trajectories were evident for a large fraction of 200-and 500-nm PEG-PS. Therefore, to further understand the unexpected rapid transport of large PEG-PS and to explain the mechanism of the contribution of PEG to improved transport, we determined the percentage of particles undergoing specific modes of transport (diffusive, hindered-diffusive, or immobile).

The greatly improved transport rates upon PEGylation, especially for larger particles, were largely due to a marked reduction in the number of immobile particles in CV mucus across all particle sizes tested. Nearly 20% of 100-nm PEG-PS were immobile, but <0.5% of 200-and 500-nm PEG-PS were immobile. In general, PEG led to an increased number of particles with greater mobility, as seen by a large shift in the transport modes from immobile to hindered-diffusion and from hindered-diffusion to diffusive. Within the size range studied here, PEGylation increased the fraction of diffusive particles between 5-and 7-fold. There was also a statistically significant increase in the percentage of diffusive particles when the particle size was increased from 100 to 200 or 500 nm. The difference in the percentage of hindered and diffusive particles between 200-and 500-nm samples was not statistically significant for both surface chemistries tested. Furthermore, PEGylation also improved the overall transport rates of similar-sized particles undergoing hindered transport for all particle sizes. At a time scale of 1 s, PEGylated particles displayed 6.0-, 99-, and 140-fold faster transport within the hindered diffusion regime than their non-PEGylated 100-, 200-, and 500-nm counterparts, respectively.

Within the hindered populations, 200-nm PEG-modified particles displayed the greatest mobility, and even 500-nm PEGylated particles moved much more rapidly than similar 100-nm particles. However, considering exclusively the diffusive population of particles, an increase in particle size reduced transport rates, and 100-nm particles exhibited the fastest transport rates for both COOH-and PEG-modified surfaces, as expected. For diffusive PEGylated particles, a reduction in size from 500 to 200 or 100 nm increased the mean Deff by 2.3-and 3.2-fold, respectively, in adequate agreement with Stokean principles that predict 2.5-and 5-fold improvements.

Viscosity of Human CV Mucus. CV mucus exhibits viscosity within the range (in the higher end) of typical human mucus secretions.

Discussion

Encapsulation of drugs and genes in nanoparticles offers the potential for direct and sustained delivery to the underlying epithelial cells in mucus-covered tissues, including the CV tract, thus minimizing systemic toxicity and degradation of the cargo therapeutics in serum. Nanoparticles must quickly traverse CV mucus layers that are up to a few hundred microns thick to reach the underlying epithelia and avoid mucus clearance mechanisms. An important role of mucus barriers is to trap foreign particles and then clear them from the body before they reach the underlying epithelia. The mucus barrier has been cited as a critical bottleneck in the treatment of a variety of diseases, and it has been widely suggested that nanoparticles are unable to efficiently traverse mucus layers, including CV mucus. For applications in CV diseases, the need for improved particle transport is further underscored by:

(i) the previous observation that polystyrene beads firmly adhere to mucin fibers in human CV secretions, rendering them completely immobile;

(ii) there is 100-to 1,000-fold reduced Deff for herpes simplex virus (d = 180 nm) in CV mucus compared with water; and

(iii) there are existing estimates of CV mucus mesh pore size of 10 to at most 200 nm from fluorescence recovery after photobleaching (FRAP) and most electron microscopy studies. The prevalent dogma in the design of nanoparticle therapeutics targeted to mucosal epithelia is that large nanoparticles, preferred for higher drug-encapsulation efficiency and favorable drug-release kinetics, are not capable of crossing mucosal barriers.

Surprisingly, we report that the transport of PEG-coated polymer particles larger than the reported CV mucus-mesh size was not significantly impeded by CV mucus. Specifically, using multiple particle tracking, which traces the motions of hundreds of individual particles with high temporal and spatial resolution, we found that size, surface chemistry, and particle concentration all critically influence the transport of particles in human CV mucus. The most surprising findings were:

(i) larger polymeric nanoparticles (up to 500 nm) with a dense polyethylene-glycol coating can diffuse through CV mucus with rates up to one-fourth as fast as they would in pure water; and

(ii) 100-nm particles moved much more slowly through CV mucus than either 200-or 500-nm particles.

The faster transport of 200-and 500-nm particles, regardless of surface chemistry (COOH or PEG), not only is contrary to the expectation that smaller particles should move faster in mucus but also directly opposes the earlier estimates of CV mucus mesh spacing. Greater steric hindrance from the mucin fiber network and elevated friction forces was expected, a priori, to result in slower transport for larger particles in CV mucus. However, we observed both greater immobile and hindered-diffusion fractions for 100-nm particles compared with either 200-or 500-nm particles for both COOH-and PEG-modified surfaces. The large fraction of 200-and 500-nm particles that underwent diffusive transport (e.g., as opposed to hindered diffusion) directly implied that the upper range of effective mesh spacing in human CV secretions must be significantly larger than earlier reports and must include a large number of pores with effective spacings substantially larger than 500 nm. This spacing is consistent with the only electron microscopic investigation in which the mucus gel was prepared by freeze substitution. With this method, the spacing between the primary fibrous elements was 500-800 nm, suggesting freeze substitution may cause minimal disturbance of the native distribution of mucin fibers. The rapid mucosal transport of 200-and 500-nm PEG-modified particles has important implications for the development of therapeutic and imaging applications in vivo. Larger nanoparticles afford substantially higher drug encapsulation efficiency, and the release of drugs from small nanoparticles (<100-200 nm) is difficult to control. The high surface-area-to-volume ratio of small nanoparticles typically leads to fast diffusion of drugs out of particles (i.e., the burst effect) within hours upon in vitro or in vivo application. As the size of drug-loaded particles increases, drug-release kinetics are usually greatly improved, and sustained release of therapeutics over days and even months can be achieved with enhanced therapeutic efficacies.

It is possible that large PEGylated nanoparticles may also transport quickly in mucus coating other entry sites into the body. Mucus coatings of the CV tract, airways of the lungs, gastrointestinal tract, nose, eyes, and epididymus all have similar components, and all possess similar rheological properties. In particular, the mucin glycoform MUC5B has been identified as the major secreted form of mucin in the mucosal layers protecting the CV tract, lungs, nose, and eye. The mucin content, 1-3% by weight, is also similar among cervical, nasal, and lung mucus. The composition of water in the aforementioned mucus types all falls within the range of 90-98%. The similar mucus composition and mucin glycoforms leads to similar rheology, characterized by log-linear shear thinning of viscosity. It should be recognized, however, that, with the exception of mucus expectorated by patients with cystic fibrosis, it remains very difficult to obtain fresh undiluted human mucus from sites other than the CV tract.

The transport of hydrophobic polystyrene particles without PEG modification was characterized by significant entrapment within and adhesion to the mucosal network, presumably because of the hydrophobic polystyrene bead-forming polyvalent bonds with hydrophobic domains distributed along mucin fibers.

However, it was not obvious, a priori, that PEG may reduce association of particles with mucus components, because high-molecular mass PEG (>10 kDa) has been shown to exhibit mucoadhesive properties involving interpenetration of the polymer with mucus fibers. Looking to nature for guidance, we noted that viruses capable of rapid transport in mucus possess surfaces that are densely coated equally with positive and negative charges, creating a hydrophilic and net-neutral shell that minimizes hydrophobic and electrostatic adhesive interactions.

However, the engineering of densely charged (average distance between charges, 5 Å) yet neutral surfaces on synthetic particles is exceedingly difficult. We hypothesized that coating particles with PEG, an uncharged hydrophilic polymer routinely used in pharmaceutics, may reduce particle-mucus adhesive interactions if the molecular mass of PEG was too low to support adhesion by polymer interpenetration. We show here that, contrary to reports of PEG as mucoadhesive, coating particles with 2-kDa PEG chains led to a greatly increased percentage of diffusive particles and up to 3 orders of magnitude faster transport.

It is unlikely that the rapid transport of PEGylated particles is due to alterations of the mucus structure, because they do not interact significantly with mucus. Instead, particles likely move in low-viscosity channels or pores within the mucus, as suggested in our earlier work on particle transport in cystic fibrosis mucus. We have recently found that PEGylated particles move much faster in cystic fibrosis mucus than non-PEGylated particles of equal size over time scales of at least 40 min and distances of at least 7.4 μm using biodegradable poly(ether-anhydride) nanoparticles [our unpublished results; the polymer has been described, suggesting that transport rates of PEGylated particles measured at short time scales correlate well with those measured at long time scales in mucus.

One possible explanation for the significant fraction of 100-nm PEG-modified particles that remain immobile in the mucosal network (whereas <0.5% of 200-and 500-nm PEG-PS are immobile) may be attributed to inadequate PEGylation of 100-nm (vs. 200-or 500-nm) particles. Smaller particles, because of a greater degree of curvature, may require higher surface density of hydrophilic PEG molecules to sufficiently shield the hydrophobic core. However, the effectiveness of the PEG shield, as measured by surface charge and resistance to avidin adsorption, appeared similar for all particles studied. Alternatively, the unexpected slower transport of 100-nm particles in the viscoelastic CV mucus gel may be partially explained by principles from size-exclusion chromatography. According to this theory, for particles of various sizes traveling in a network with heterogeneous pore sizes, smaller particles can access a greater number of small pores or pockets in the gel, resulting in an overall reduced transport rate over long distances because of the greatly increased tortuosity of their average path.

Larger particles that are unable to diffuse into small pores move instead in less-restricted low-viscosity channels, with much larger mesh spacing. It seems unlikely, however, that this hypothesis can be reconciled with the previous observation that viruses <55 nm in diameter can diffuse basically unhindered in CV mucus. We were able to rule out aggregation as a potential explanation for the slower transport of 100-nm particles for several reasons:

(i) particles were not aggregated before addition to mucus (or glycerol; results not shown), as measured by dynamic light scattering;

(ii) high particle monodispersity was observed in both glycerol and mucus, where polydispersity is expected for aggregated particles;

(iii) we found that measured transport rates of particles in glycerol correctly reflect its viscosity based on the Stokes-Einstein equation; and

(iv) heavily PEGylated nanoparticles are highly resistant to aggregation.

A number of reports have examined particle size and transport or cellular uptake in mucosal environments; however, none has reported observations of smaller particles moving more slowly than larger particles. The majority of studies compared particle sizes spanning orders of magnitude and concluded that smaller particles move faster.

It is difficult to directly compare these studies to the results reported here, given the large deviation in the range of particle sizes previously studied and the different types of mucus tested.

Others have reported that permeability values decreased sharply as the particle size was increased from 100 to 300 nm in synthetic gastric mucin gels or rat gastrointestinal mucosa. It remains unknown whether the discrepancy between these findings and ours is a consequence of differences in the biophysical structure of the mucin fiber networks (i.e., synthetic formulations vs. physiological secretions), the types of mucus being compared, and/or collection and handling methods used.

Differences between our study and the previous report by Cone and coworkers led us to another important finding. Specifically, we found that a significant number of polystyrene particles were able to move in human cervical mucus, whereas Olmsted et al. reported that all particles were immobile. The principal differences between the two studies may be related to the concentration of particles used. The experiments performed here used diluted COOH-PS and PEG-PS, whereas the Olmsted study used more concentrated COOH-PS. We found that the addition of high concentrations of COOH-PS particles collapsed mucus fibers into bundles (data not shown) in a manner similar to that observed in the Olmsted study.

In the latter case, the concentrated particle solution likely contains a sufficient number of particles to impart a hydrophobic force capable of affecting the mucosal network structure. Once the mucin fibers collapse around the particles, there are sufficient hydrophobic interactions to stabilize the particles, resulting in complete retardation of transport. The observation that the concentration of particles may critically affect the transport in mucus warrants further study. By eliminating the hydrophobic interactions between mucin fibers and hydrophobic polystyrene core, PEGylation may allow delivery of rapidly moving particles to the mucosa at higher concentrations than otherwise possible with uncoated particles, potentially increasing the concentration of therapeutics that can be delivered to the mucosal surfaces of the body.

Summary

Unexpectedly, large (200-to 500-nm) particles transport much more rapidly than 100-nm particles in human CV mucus. This finding should strongly encourage the commercial development of new nanoparticle-based drug delivery systems for the CV tract and potentially other mucosal surfaces, because drug-delivery kinetics and loading efficiency are vastly improved as particle diameter increases. Our study also suggests that a larger effective mucus-mesh size exists for CV mucus than previously reported. Particle concentration may also play an important role in particle transport across mucosal barriers and, therefore, should be studied further. The design of particles with improved physical (e.g., size) and chemical (e.g., surface chemistry) properties may lead to improved drug delivery to the CV tract by enhancing the ability of drug-delivery systems to cross the mucus barrier.

SUMMARY

Enormous progress is being made in understanding the molecular basis of endocrine-related cancer, and this brings great potential to design improved therapeutic strategies. Although the pharmaceutical industry prefers to develop small-molecule anticancer agents that can be administered to patients orally (very convenient to use), macro-molecular drugs and delivery systems, including antibodies, proteins and polymer conjugates, are establishing their niche in modern chemotherapy. It is now universally agreed that combination approaches, perhaps involving small molecules (endocrine and chemotherapy), macromolecular drugs such as antibodies, and DDS, including polymer therapeutics, will probably be required to increase therapeutic index and circumvent all routes to resistance.

6

Nanoparticles in the Treatment of Cancer

In ancient Greek 'Nano' means dwarf. Nanotechnology is the creation and utilization of materials, devices, and systems through the control of matter on the nanometer-length scale, i.e. at the level of atoms, molecules, and supramolecular structures. These technologies have been applied to improve drug delivery and to overcome some of the problems of drug delivery for cancer treatment. Several nanobiotechnologies mostly based on nanoparticles, have been used to facilitate drug delivery in cancer. The magic of nanoparticles mesmerize everyone because of their multifunctional character and they have given us hope for the recovery from this disease. Although we are practicing better drug delivery paths into the body, we ultimately seek more accurate protocols to eradicate cancer from our society. This review focuses on progress in treatment of cancer through delivery of anticancer agents via nanoparticles. In addition, it pays attention to development of different types of nanoparticles for cancer drug delivery.

CANCER CASES

Cancer in Our Society

With more than 10 million new cases every year, cancer has become one of the most devastating diseases worldwide. In 2000, it has been reported by The World Health Organization (WHO), malignant tumors were responsible for 12 per cent of the nearly 56 million deaths worldwide from all causes.

Over 22 million people in the world were treated for cancer in 2000, representing an increase of approximately 19 percent in incidence (cases) and 18 percent in mortality since 1990. In many countries, more than a quarter of deaths are attributable to cancer.

THE INCIDENCE OF CANCER

In 2000, 5.3 million men and 4.7 million women developed a malignant tumor and altogether 6.2 million died from the disease. The report also reveals that cancer has emerged as a major public health problem in developing countries, matching its effect in industrialized nations.

The predicted sharp increase in new cases from 10 million new cases globally in 2000, to 15 million in 2020 9will mainly be due to steadily ageing populations in both developed and developing countries and also to current trends in smoking prevalence and the growing adoption of unhealthy lifestyles.

Projected Growth of Cancer in the Future

In 2005, a total of 7.6million people died of cancer. More than 11 million people are diagnosed with cancer every year. It is estimated that there will be 16 million new cases every year by 2020. Cancer causes 7 million deaths every year or 12.5% of deaths worldwide.

Some 60% of all these new cases will occur in the less developed parts of the world. Global cancer rates are expected to increase 50 percent by the year 2020, according to the latest report from the International Agency for Research on Cancer (IARC), a branch of the World Health Organization.

Structure and Functional Properties of Nanoparticles

A nanometer is one-billionth of a meter (10-9 m); a sheet of paper is about 100,000 nanometers thick. These nanoparticles give us the ability to see cells and molecules that we otherwise cannot detect through conventional imaging. The ability to pick up what happens in the cell, to monitor therapeutic intervention and to see when a cancer cell is mortally wounded or is actually activated is critical for the successful diagnosis and treatment of this disease.

For drug delivery in cancer we have "Nano scale devices". Nanoscale devices are 102 to 104 times smaller than human cells but are similar in size to large biomolecules such as enzymes and receptors.

Nanoscale devices smaller than 50 nm can easily enter most cells, and those smaller than 20 nm can move out of blood vessels as they circulate through the body. Nanodevices are suitable to serve as customized, targeted drug delivery vehicles to carry large doses of chemotherapeutic agents or therapeutic genes into malignant cells while sparing healthy cells.

According to The National Cancer Institute, Nanoparticulate technology can prove to be very useful in cancer therapy allowing for effective and targeted drug delivery by overcoming the many biological, biophysical and biomedical barriers that the body stages against a standard intervention such as the administration of drugs or contrast agents.

Nanoscale constructs can serve as customizable, targeted drug delivery vehicles capable of ferrying large doses of chemotherapeutic agents or therapeutic genes into malignant cells while sparing healthy cells, greatly reducing or eliminating the often unpalatable side effects that accompany many current cancer therapies. Several nanotechnological approaches have been used to improve delivery of chemotherapeutic agents to cancer cells with the goal of minimizing toxic effects on healthy tissues while maintaining antitumor efficacy. Some nanoscale delivery devices, such as dendrimers (spherical, branched polymers), silica-coated micelles, ceramic nanoparticles, and cross linked liposomes can be targeted to cancer cells. This increase the selectivity of drugs towards cancer cells can and will reduce the toxicity to normal tissue.

BIOMEDICAL NANOPARTICLES

Although the number of different type of nanoparticles is increasing rapidly, most can be classified into two major types. Particles that contain organic molecules as a major building material and those that use inorganic elements, usually metals, as a core

- Inorganic nanoparticles
- Organic nanoparticles

Liposomes, dendrimers, carbon nanotubes, emulsions, and other polymers are a large and well-established group of organic particles. Use of these organic nanoparticles has already produced exciting results. Liposomes are being used as vehicles for drug delivery in different human tumors, including breast cancer. Dendrimers, used in MRI as contrast agents, have aided visualisation of various pathological processes. Conjugated with pharmacological agents and targeting molecules, organic nanovectors are potent vehicles for drug delivery and selective imaging of different human cancers. Most inorganic nanoparticles share the same basic structure. This consists of a central core that defines the fluorescence, optical, magnetic, and electronic properties of the particle, with a protective organic coating on the surface. This outside layer protects the core from degradation in a physiologically aggressive environment and can form electrostatic or covalent bonds, or both, with positively charged agents and biomolecules that have basic functional groups such as amines and thiols. Several research groups have successfully linked fluorescent nanoparticles to peptides, proteins, and oligonucleotides.

MULTIFUNCTIONAL NANOPARTICLES

Nanoparticles have a further advantage over larger microparticles, because they are better suited for intravenous (i.v.) delivery. The smallest capillaries in the body are 5–6 mm in diameter. The size of particles being distributed into the bloodstream must be significantly smaller than 5 mm, without forming aggregates, to ensure that the particles do not form an embolism. Nanoparticles can be used to deliver hydrophilic drugs, hydrophobic drugs, proteins, vaccines, biological macromolecules, etc. They can be formulated for targeted delivery to the lymphatic system, brain, arterial walls, lungs, liver, spleen, or made for long-term systemic circulation. Therefore, numerous protocols exist for synthesizing nanoparticles based on the type of drug used and the desired delivery route. Once a protocol is chosen, the parameters must be tailored to create the best possible characteristics for the nanoparticles.

Four of the most important characteristics of nanoparticles are their size, encapsulation efficiency, zeta potential (surface charge), and release characteristics. Different nanoparticles have been discussed below.

Lipid/Polymer Nanoparticles

Positively charged lipid-based nanoparticles are known to trigger strong immune responses when injected into the body. This can be problematic when attempting to use this type of nanoparticle as a drug delivery vehicle. Lipid-based cationic nanoparticles are a new promising option for tumor therapy, because they display enhanced binding and uptake at the neo-angiogenic endothelial cells, which a tumor needs for its nutrition and growth. By loading suitable cytotoxic compounds to the cationic carrier, the tumor endothelial and consequently also the tumor itself can be destroyed. For the development of such novel anti-tumor agents, the control of drug loading and drug release from the carrier matrix is essential. Structural investigation of drug/lipid membranes may give valuable information about the organization of drugs in lipid matrices.

Screening of different matrices for a given drug may be useful for fast and efficient optimization of drug/lipid combinations in pharmaceutical development. In a new therapeutic approach, targeted drug delivery is performed not to the tumor itself, but to the neo-angiogenic blood vessels that the tumor stimulates to grow for its nutrition. This procedure is based on the observation that cationic liposomes show enhanced binding and uptake at tumor endothelial cells. In this context Munich Biotech AG has developed a series of cationic, lipid based, nanoparticulate agents for tumor therapy and diagnosis. The therapeutic agents consist of a cytotoxic compound, such as Paclitaxel, which is loaded into the lipid matrix of the cationic carrier. For efficient development of such pharmaceutical formulations, it is useful to obtain an insight into the physico-chemical constraints of drug loading and drug release from the lipid matrix.

Structural investigation of drug/lipid membranes, for example by X-ray scattering techniques, can give valuable information about the organization of a drug in the membrane, and it can help to optimize a lipid matrix with respect to its solubilizing potency of a given drug. In this work, attention was given to the organization of Paclitaxel in matrices of cationic and zwitterionic lipid membranes. Polymeric nanoparticle, are stable and non-phototoxic upon systemic administration. Upon cellular internalization, the photosensitizer is released from the nanoparticle and becomes highly phototoxic. Irradiation with visible light results in cell-specific killing of several cancer cell lines.

Gold / Magnetic Nanoparticles

In practice, gold nanoparticles are the most commonly used nanoparticles for diagnostics and drug delivery. The unique chemical properties of colloidal gold make it a promising targeted delivery approach for drugs or gene specific cells. Gold and silica composite nanoparticles have been investigated as nanobullets for cancer. Researchers are also using magnetic nanoparticles for cancer drug delivery. The use of magnetic nanoparticles in cell biology was first proposed in the early 1990s, and their use has made the separation of cells or molecules such as proteins, peptides and DNA considerably easier.

In medicine, nanoparticles first found use in the diagnosis of tumors in the liver and spleen using magnetic resonance tomography. In cancer therapy a major difficulty is to destroy tumor cells without harming the normal tissue. Radiotherapy attempts to focus irradiation on the tumor, but nevertheless damages healthy tissue which cannot always be protected in the desired way. Magnetic drug targeting employing nanoparticles as the carrier is a promising cancer treatment avoiding side effects of conventional chemotherapy. There is also a very significant role of hyperthermia in cancer drug delivery. There is increasing evidence that hyperthermia at 40–43°C enhances the uptake of therapeutic agents into cancer cells and provides an opportunity for improved targeted drug delivery. Using nanoparticles (NPs) for drug delivery of anticancer agents has significant advantages such as the ability to target specific locations in the body, the reduction of the overall quantity of drug used, and the potential to reduce the concentration of the drug at non target sites resulting in fewer unpleasant side effects.

Furthermore, certain type of nanoparticles showed some interesting capacity to reverse multi drug resistance (MDR) which is a major problem in chemotherapy. The use of nanoparticles as drug delivery vehicles for anticancer therapeutics has great potential to revolutionise the future of cancer therapy. As tumor architecture causes nanoparticles to preferentially accumulate at the tumor site, their use as drug delivery vectors results in the localization of a greater amount of the drug load at the tumor site; thus improving cancer therapy and reducing the harmful nonspecific side effects of chemotherapeutics. In addition, formulation of these nanoparticles with imaging contrast agents provides a very efficient system for cancer diagnostics.

Virus Based Nanoparticles

In the latest research development virus-based nano-particles are being extensively investigated for nanobiotechnology applications. Viruses have long been envisaged as nanoparticle vectors suitable for drug delivery, vaccines, and gene therapy. Recently, viruses have been explored as nano-containers for specific targeting applications. However these systems typically require modification of the virus surface using chemical or genetic means to achieve tumor-specific delivery. The latest technology developed engineered virus (nanoparticles) for cancer treatment. Viruses by their extraordinarily nature are well-defined nanoparticles, and several teams of investigators are taking a cue from nature and developing non-infectious, engineered viral nanoparticles for use as multifunctional nanoscale devices.

The plant virus known as (CPMV) cowpea mosaic virus (CPMV and FHV are among the smallest viruses with diverse nanostructures extensively investigated, and are strategically more suitable for rapid dispersal within tumors than adenoviruses three times their size) has become a research favorite, in large part because it is relatively easy to produce in large amounts, and the virus is benign to humans and other animals.

In addition, researchers have developed methods of altering the virus's coat protein to give it chemical functionality that might be useful for adding targeting and drug delivery capabilities to these nanoparticles. Now, there's another reason to study CPMV particles as potential biomedical nanodevices. M. Manchester, M.G. Finn, and their colleagues at the Scripps Research Institute have shown that CPMV nanoparticles can pass intact through the stomach's hostile environment and be taken into the bloodstream through the intestines.

As a result, CMPV nanoparticles could provide a means of administering anticancer drugs and tumor imaging agents orally, rather than by injection. This work appeared in the journal Virology. In most studies, researchers produce CPMV nanoparticles using a system that makes just the proteins that the virus uses to make its outer shell – these proteins self-assemble to make the virus's shell. But to learn what would happen to CPMV particles as they pass through the digestive system, the researchers used the fully formed virus, complete with its RNA genetic material. Having the RNA present allowed the investigators to use PCR-based technology to detect a very small number of particles no matter what part of the body they reached. Indeed, after feeding mice cowpea leaves infected with the virus, the investigators found virus particles distribute widely throughout the animal's bodies.

Subsequent studies using analytical techniques to detect the virus coat proteins confirmed that the virus particle, and not just its genetic material, had passed through the stomach, been absorbed through the intestines, and distributed itself throughout the animal. Nearly identical results were obtained when the virus was injected directly into the bloodstream of the test animals, supporting the idea that virus particles were able to pass through the intestines unaltered. In vitro experiments also showed that engineered CPMV particles are stable in conditions that mimic the acidic conditions of the stomach. Taken together, these data sets support the notion that engineered, synthetic plant virus particles could prove useful in delivering drugs and imaging contrast agents to tumors. Previous work by the Manchester and Finn groups has already shown that it is possible to attach tumor-targeting molecules to the surface of engineered viral nanoparticles and to load various drug-type molecules into the interior of the virus particles.

A research team from Yonsei University uses a genetically-engineered form of the adenovirus, which normally causes colds. The adenovirus was implanted with a human gene that is related to the production of relaxin, a hormone associated with pregnancy. When injected into cancerous tumors, the virus quickly multiplies in the cancer cells and kills them. The new adenovirus can target only cancer cells and does not harm normal cells.

Dry Powder Aerosol

An approach regarding drug delivery has been taken by Dr. Lobenberg, University of Alberta, i.e. a lung cancer treatment using nanoparticles in dry powder aerosol form. Drug-loaded nanoparticles carried by dry powders showed a concentration related increased cytotoxicity in vitro. This study supports the approach of local lung cancer treatment using nanoparticles as a drug delivery vector. The development of inhalable nanoparticles loaded with bioactive molecules is a new delivery platform which can allow targeting of lung specific diseases in the future. Loebenberg explained that the drug sits in powder form in the inhaler, which is similar to the device that asthmatics use.

Nanomedicine

When we think about nanomedicine then the first thing that comes to our mind is exactly why nanomedicine?

One of the main goals of nanomedicine is to create medically useful nanodevices that can function inside the body. Additionally, nanomedicine will have an impact on the key challenges in cancer therapy such as localized drug delivery and specific targeting. Among the recently developed nanomedicine and nanodevices, quantum dots, nanowires, nanotubes, nanocantilevers, nanopores, nanoshells and nanoparticles are potentially the most useful for treating different types of cancer. Nanoparticles can be in the form of nanospheres (matrix systems in which drugs are dispersed throughout the particle) and nanocapsules (where the drug is confined in an aqueous or oily cavity surrounded by a single polymeric membrane). Nanomedicines are a recent off-shoot of the application of nanotechnology to medical and pharmaceutical challenges, but have in fact been around for much longer in the guise of drug delivery systems. Nanomedicines that facilitate uptake and transport of therapeutically active molecules ('delivery systems') tend to be based on supramolecular assemblies of drug and functional carrier materials. The use of nanomedicines facilitates the creation of dose differentials between the site of the disease and the rest of the body, thus maximizing the therapeutic effect while minimizing non-specific side-effects. Nanomedicine, the use of nanometer-sized particles and systems to detect and treat diseases at the molecular level plays an essential role in achieving the federal governments stated goal of eliminating suffering and death from cancer, the second leading cause of death in the United States, by 2015.

HERBAL NANOPARTICLES FOR CANCER TREATMENT

The whole world is practicing herbal medicine to avoid maximum side effects and for better treatment. The science of Ayurveda is supposed to add a step on to curative aspects of cancers. There are many herbs like Aswagandha, Amla, Basil, Rakta vrntaka (Tomato), Neem, Turmeric etc with anticancerous properties. Antioxidants play an important role in mitigating the damaging effects of oxidative stress on cells. Lycopene, a carotenoid, has received considerable scientific interest in recent years. They have demonstrated a very special role in the curing of cancer. In the past several years, two lines of emerging evidence have supported a role for lycopene in the prevention of certain malignancies, especially prostate cancer. Tomato is a rich source of lycopene. The first, antioxidant properties of lycopene (Lycopersicon esculentum) have been established. Given the relatively high concentrations of lycopene in the tissues of many individuals, and the potential role of oxidative stress in the formation or progression of cancers, a potential anticancer influence of lycopene has been hypothesized. Secondly, a number of epidemiologic studies have suggested that individuals with a relatively high intake of lycopene, particularly from tomato products, have a lower risk of prostate cancer. In the future, the concept of herbal nanoparticles for cancer drug delivery may also fascinate some potential research groups and potentially create attention-grabbing results.

DEVELOPMENT AND COMMERCIALIZATION OF NANOMATERIALS

Drug delivery techniques were established to deliver or control the amount, rate and, sometimes location of a drug in the body to optimize its therapeutic effect, convenience and dose. Combining a well established drug formulation with a new delivery system is a relatively low risk activity and can be used to enhance a company's product portfolio by extending the drug's commercial life-cycle. Although not exhausting, this is a representative selection reflecting current industrial trends. Most companies are developing pharmaceutical applications, mainly for drug delivery. Most major and established pharmaceutical companies have internal research programs on drug delivery that are on formulations or dispersions containing components down to nano sizes. With the total global investment in nanotechnologies currently at 5 billion, the global market is estimated to reach over 1 trillion by 2011-2015. Nano and Micro technologies are part of the latest advanced solutions and new paradigm for decreasing the discovery and development time for new drugs and potentially reducing the development costs.

THE ROLE OF NANOPARTICLES IN CANCER DRUG DELIVERY

Nanoparticles and other nanostructures appear to hold greatIn experimental studies, primarily in animal models, nanoparticles appear to be able to selectively deliver high concentrations of antitumour drugs to tumor cells. The high concentrations of toxic agents seem to persist for long periods within tumor cells and have more potent antitumour effects and less toxicity than their systematically administered counterparts. Nanoparticles are much more successful at delivering anticancer agents during drug delivery to cancer cells or tissues.

Cancer disease challenging nanoparticles may be defined as being submicronic (< 1 μm) colloidal systems generally, but not necessarily, made of polymers (biodegradable or not). According to the process used for the preparation of the nanoparticles, nanospheres or nanocapsules can be obtained. Unlike nanospheres (matrix systems in which the drug is dispersed throughout the particles), nanocapsules are vesicular systems in which the drug is confined to an aqueous or oily cavity surrounded by a single polymeric membrane. Nanocapsules may, thus, be considered as a 'reservoir' system. If designed appropriately, it may act as a drug vehicle able to target tumor tissues or cells, to a certain extent, while protecting the drug from premature inactivation during its transport. Indeed, at the tumor level, the accumulation mechanism of intravenously injected nanoparticles relies on a passive diffusion or convection across the leaky, hyperpermeable tumor vasculature. The uptake can also result from a specific recognition in the case of ligand decorated nanoparticles ('active targeting'). Understanding and experience from other technologies such as Nanotechnology, Advanced Polymer Chemistry, and Electronic Engineering, are being brought together in developing novel methods of drug delivery.

The current focus in development of cancer therapies is on targeted drug delivery to provide therapeutic concentrations of anticancer agents at the site of action and to spare the normal tissues. Cancer drug delivery is no longer simply packaging the drug in new formulations for unlike routes of delivery.

Targeted drug delivery to tumors can increase the selectivity for killing cancer cells, decrease the peripheral/systemic toxicity and can permit a dose escalation. So targeted drug delivery will be more advantageous. These days drug delivery using micro/nano particles has been shown to have great potentials for achieving controlled and targeted therapeutic effects. The carrier particles have specific transportation and extravasation behaviors determined by their chemical structure, size, and surface properties etc. These characteristics are vital for the pharmacokinetics and pharmacodynamics of drugs being carried.

To reach cancer cells in a tumor, a blood borne therapeutic molecule or cell must make its ways into the blood vessels of the tumor and across the vessel wall into interstitium, and finally migrate through the interstitium. For a molecule of given size, charge, and configuration, each of these transport processes may involve diffusion and convection. In the year 2002, there was a very fascinating article published in Science entitled "Nanoparticles Cut Tumors' Supply Lines". In which, hungry tumors need new blood vessels for sustenance to deliver the goods. Cancer researchers have spent years working to starve tumors by blocking this blood vessel growth, or angiogenesis, with mixed success. The researchers packed a tiny particle with a gene that forces blood vessel cells to self-destruct, then they "mailed" the particle to blood vessels feeding tumors in mice. This is the latest achievement in the field of cancer treatment which is giving new hope for cancer patients who are suffering from angiogenesis.

Targeted drug delivery is an invaluable need in pharmacology. Such an approach is particularly important in tumor therapy as the compounds are very toxic, and if they act on cells other than tumor cells, severe side effects are encountered. Any means that enables the increase of the ratio of the drug, which is delivered to the target site, will help to reduce such side effects.

DETECTION AND CURE WITH NANODEVICES

"Smart" dynamic nanoplatforms have the potential to change the way cancer is diagnosed, treated, and prevented. There are two basic approaches for creating nanodevices. Scientists refer to these methods as the top-down approach and the bottom-up approach. The top-down approach involves molding or etching materials into smaller components. This approach has traditionally been used in making parts for computers and electronics. The bottom-up approach involves assembling structures atom-by-atom or molecule-by-molecule, and may prove useful in manufacturing devices used in medicine.

Most animal cells are 10,000 to 20,000 nanometers in diameter. This means that nanoscale devices (less than 100 nanometers) can enter cells and the organelles inside them can interact with DNA and proteins. Tools developed through nanotechnology may be able to detect disease in a very small amount of cells or tissue.

They may also be able to enter and monitor cells within a living body. In order to successfully detect cancer at its earliest stages, scientists must be able to detect molecular changes even when they occur only in a small percentage of cells. This means the necessary tools must be extremely sensitive. The potential for nanostructures to enter and analyze single cells suggests they could meet this need.

Cantilevers

Nanoscaled cantilevers like springs are being developed using electron-beam lithography for an ultra sensitive bioassay. The flexible nature of the technology has the potential to offer high-throughput detection of proteins,

DNA and RNA for a broad range of applications ranging from disease diagnosis to biological weapons detection. Through e-beam lithography and lift-off processes, arrays of nano-cantilevers have been fabricated. These arrays can be used as non-invasive and ultra-sensitive bio-assays, and provide an opportunity to increase the sensitivity of detection of tumor-associated antigens with a smaller sample size and at much earlier stages of disease progression compared to current medical diagnostic technologies. Cantilevers can improve cancer detection and diagnosis. These tiny levers, which are anchored at one end, can be engineered to bind to molecules that represent some of the changes associated with cancer. They may bind to altered DNA sequences or proteins that are present in certain types of cancer. When these molecules bind to the cantilevers, surface tension changes, causing the cantilevers to bend. By monitoring the bending of the cantilevers, scientists can tell whether molecules are present. Scientists hope this property will prove effective when cancer-associated molecules are present even in very low concentrations-making cantilevers a potential tool for detecting cancer in its early stages.

Nanopores

Another interesting nanodevice is the nanopore. Improved methods of reading the genetic code will help researchers detect errors in genes that may contribute to cancer. Scientists believe nanopores, tiny holes that allow DNA to pass through one strand at a time, will make DNA sequencing more efficient. As DNA passes through a nanopore, scientists can monitor the shape and electrical properties of each base, or letter, on the strand. Because these properties are unique for each of the four bases that make up the genetic code, scientists can use the passage of DNA through a nanopore to decipher the encoded information, including errors in the code known to be associated with cancer.

Nanotubes

Another nanodevice that will help identify DNA changes associated with cancer is the nanotube. Nanotubes are carbon rods about half the diameter of a molecule of DNA that can not only can detect the presence of altered genes, but they may help researchers pinpoint the exact location of those changes. Carbon nanotubes (CNTs) are remarkable solid state nanomaterials due to their unique electrical and mechanical properties. The electronic properties of nanotubes combined with biological molecules such as proteins could make miniature devices for biological sensing applications.

The research of carbon nanotube functionalization has intensified due to their great potential for biomedical and biotechnological applications. Organic modification of carbon nanotubes generate multiple sites for the attachment of bioactive molecules, and the modified nanotube could be used as a biosensor or a novel delivery system. Carbon Nanotubes Target Tumors in the first experiment of its kind Investigators at the Center for Cancer Nanotechnology Response (CCNE-TR), based at Stanford University. Experiments have shown that single-walled carbon nanotubes (SWCNTs) wrapped in poly(ethylene glycol), or PEG, can successfully target tumors in living animals.

Quantum Dots (QDs)

Quantum dots are unique in their far reaching possibilities in many avenues of medicine. A QD is a fluorescent nanoparticle that has potential to be used as a sensitive probe for screening cancer markers in fluids, as a specific label for classifying tissue biopsies and as a high resolution contrast agent for medical imaging, which is capable of detecting even the smallest of tumors. These particles have the unique ability to be sensitively detected on a wide range of length scales, from macroscale visualization, down to atomic resolution using electron microscopy. Using Quantum dots (QDs), the drug delivery particles are injected in to blood stream until they find the cancer cells, to which the antibodies adhere. Infrared light shining on the suspected cancer site penetrates the tissues and cause the quantum dots to radiate photons.

The photons pinpoint the cancer cell's location and also cause the release of the Taxol (an anticancerous drug), which can then attack and kill the cancer cells. Quantum dots are tiny crystals that glow when stimulated by ultraviolet light. The wavelength, or color, of the light depends on the size of the crystal. Latex beads filled with these crystals can be designed to bind to specific DNA sequences. By combining different sized quantum dots within a single bead, scientists can create probes that release distinct colors and intensities of light. When the crystals are stimulated by UV light, each bead emits light that serves as a sort of spectral bar code, identifying a particular region of DNA. The diversity of quantum dots will allow scientists to create many unique labels, which can identify numerous regions of DNA simultaneously. This will be important in the detection of cancer, which results from the accumulation of many different changes within a cell. Another advantage of quantum dots is that they can be used in the body, eliminating the need for biopsy.

Nanoshells

Nanoshells are layered colloids with a nonconducting nanoparticle core covered by a thin metal shell, whose thickness can be changed to precisely tune the plasmon resonance. Proteins that bind only with tumor cells can be attached to the surface, creating tumor-seeking nanoparticles. By tuning the shells to strongly absorb 820 nm NIR light, where optical transmission through body tissue is optimal and harmless, low-power extracorporeally applied laser light shone at the patient induces a response signal from injected nanoshells clustered around a tumor. Increasing the laser power to a still moderately low exposure heats the nanoshells just enough to destroy the tumor without harming healthy tissue. On exposure to 35 W/cm^2 NIR light, human breast carcinoma cells incubated with nanoshells in vitro undergo photothermally induced morbidity. Cells without nanoshells display no loss in viability. Likewise, in vivo studies under magnetic resonance guidance reveal that exposure to low-dose (4 W/cm^2) NIR light in solid tumors treated with nanoshells incur a temperature increase of 37.4±6.6°C within 4-6 minutes. The tissue displays coagulation, cell shrinkage, and loss of nuclear staining, indicating irreversible thermal damage. Controls treated without nanoshells demonstrated significantly lower temperatures and appeared undamaged. Miniscule beads coated with gold are also Nanoshells. By manipulating the thickness of the layers making up the nanoshells, scientists can design these beads to absorb specific wavelengths of light. The most useful nanoshells are those that absorb near-infrared light, which can easily penetrate several centimeters of human tissue. The absorption of light by the nanoshells creates an intense heat that is lethal to cells. Researchers can already link nanoshells to antibodies that recognize cancer cells. Scientists envision letting these nanoshells seek out their cancerous targets, then applying near-infrared light. In laboratory cultures, the heat generated by the light-absorbing nanoshells has successfully killed tumor cells while leaving neighboring cells intact. To achieve tumor-targeted drug delivery, nanoparticle systems must address technical and biological concerns that influence their distribution.

Dendrimers

Highly branched, monodisperse macromolecules (Hyperbranched molecules) or "Dendrimers" were discovered in the early 1980's by D. Tomalia and co-workers. Dendrimers are a new class of polymeric materials. They have potential to link treatment with detection and diagnosis. Dendrimers are man-made molecules about the size of an average protein, and have a branched shape. This shape gives them vast amounts of surface area to which scientists can attach therapeutic agents or other biologically active molecules.

The structure of these materials has a great impact on their physical and chemical properties. As a result of their unique behavior dendrimers are suitable for a wide range of biomedical and industrial applications. Dendrimers are going to be very helpful in cancer treatment. Dendrimers can act as carriers, called vectors in gene therapy. Vectors transfer genes through the cell membrane into the nucleus. Currently liposomes and genetically engineered viruses have been mainly used for this purpose. The unique properties of dendrimers, such as their high degree of branching, mutivalency, globular architecture and well defined molecular weight, make them promising new scaffolds for drug delivery. Recent progress has been made in the application of biocompatible dendrimers to cancer treatment, including their use as delivery systems for potent anticancer drugs such as cisplatin and doxorubicin, as wall as agents for both boron neutron capture therapy and photodynamics therapy. Although the additional effort required for the stepwise synthesis of large dendrimers means that these molecules must possess distinct advantages over their linear polymer analogs to be useful in practical terms. Recent research has shown that dendrimers do indeed have many unique features that warrant further exploration in drug discovery.

Biodegradable Hydrogel

One of the latest approaches towards drug delivery uses hydrogels. Hydrogels can be used in various biomedical applications such as drug delivery systems, biosensors, contact lenses, catheters, and wound dressings. Hydrogels are three-dimensional, hydrophilic, polymeric networks capable of imbibing large amounts of water or biological fluids. The networks are composed of homopolymers or copolymers, and are insoluble due to the presence of chemical crosslinks (tie-points, junctions), or physical crosslinks, such as entanglements or crystallites. Hydrogels exhibit a thermodynamic compatibility with water, which allows them to swell in aqueous media. They are used to regulate drug release in reservoir-based, controlled release systems or as carriers in swellable and swelling-controlled release devices. Researchers are using biodegradable hydrogels for cancer treatment.

7

Nanocarriers for the Drug Delivery for Cancer Therapy

Nanotechnology is expected to have a dramatic impact on medicine. The application of nanotechnology for treatment, diagnosis, monitoring, and control of biological systems is now often referred to as nanomedicine. Among many possible applications of nanotechnology in medicine, the use of various nanomaterials as pharmaceutical delivery systems for drugs, DNA, and imaging agents has gained increasing attention. Many varieties of nanoparticles are available, such as different polymeric and metal nanoparticles, liposomes, niosomes, solid lipid particles, micelles, quantum dots, dendrimers, microcapsules, cells, cell ghosts, lipoproteins, and different nanoassemblies.

The paradigm of using nanoparticulate pharmaceutical carriers to enhance the in vivo efficiency of many drugs, anticancer drugs first of all, has well established itself over the past decade, in both pharmaceutical research and the clinical setting. Numerous nanoparticle-based drug delivery and drug targeting systems are currently developed or under development. Their use aims to minimize drug degradation and inactivation upon administration, prevent undesirable side effects, and increase drug bioavailability and the fraction of drug delivered in the pathological area. In general, pharmaceutical drug carriers, especially those used for parenteral administration, are expected to be biodegradable, easy, and reasonably cheap to prepare; to have a small particle size; to possess a high loading capacity; to demonstrate prolonged circulation; and, ideally, to specifically or nonspecifically accumulate in required sites in the body.

Some time ago, it was found that high-molecular-weight (40 kDa or higher), long-circulating macromolecules as well as various long-circulating nanoparticulate pharmaceutical carriers are capable of spontaneous accumulations in various pathological sites, such as solid tumors and infarcted areas, via the so-called enhanced permeability and retention (EPR) effect. This effect is based on the fact that pathological vasculature, unlike vasculature of normal healthy tissues, is "leaky"-that is, penetrable for large molecules and even for small particles-which allows for their extravasation and accumulation in an interstitial tumor space. Such accumulation is additionally facilitated by the virtual lack of a lymphatic system, responsible for the drainage of macromolecules from normal tissues, in many tumors. It has been found that the effective pore size in the endothelial lining of the blood vessels in most peripheral human tumors ranges from 200 nm to 600 nm in diameter, and the EPR effect allows for passive targeting to tumors based on the cutoff size of the leaky vasculature.

We will illustrate here the large family of pharmaceutical nanocarriers with some examples. Among particulate drug carriers, liposomes, micelles, and polymeric nanoparticles are the most extensively studied and possess the most suitable characteristics for encapsulation of many drugs, genes, and diagnostic (imaging) agents. These drug carriers as well as any other pharmaceutical nanocarriers can be surface modified by a variety of different moieties to impart them with certain properties and functionalities. These functionalities are expected to provide nanocarriers:

(1) prolonged circulation in the blood and ability to accumulate in various pathological areas (eg, solid tumors) via the EPR effect (protective polymeric coating with polyethylene glycol [PEG] is frequently used for this purpose);
(2) the ability to specifically recognize and bind target tissues or cells via the surface-attached specific ligand (monoclonal antibodies as well as their Fab fragments and some other moieties, eg, folate or transferrin, are used for this purpose);
(3) the ability to respond to local stimuli characteristic of the pathological site by, for example, releasing an entrapped drug or specifically acting on cellular membranes under the abnormal pH or temperature in disease sites (this property could be provided by surface-attached pH- or temperature-sensitive components); and
(4) the ability to penetrate inside cells bypassing lysosomal degradation for efficient targeting of intracellular drug targets (for this purpose, the surface of nanocarriers is additionally modified by cell-penetrating peptides). These are just the most evident examples. Some other specific properties can also be listed, such as an attachment of diagnostic moieties. Even the use of individual functionalities is already associated with highly positive clinical outcome; the success of Doxil, doxorubicin

in a long-circulating PEG-coated liposome, is a good example. Patient research showed the impressive effect of doxorubicin in PEG liposomes against metastatic breast carcinoma, unresectable hepatocellular carcinoma, cutaneous T-cell lymphoma, sarcoma, squamous cell cancer of the head and neck, and ovarian cancer. Liposomal lurtotecan was found to be effective in patients with topotecan-resistant ovarian cancer.

Among the most popular and well-investigated drug carriers are liposomes (mainly, for the delivery of water-soluble drugs) and micelles (for the delivery of poorly soluble drugs). Liposomes are artificial phospholipid vesicles that vary in size from 50 to 1000 nm and can be loaded with a variety of water-soluble drugs (into their inner aqueous compartment) and sometimes even with water-insoluble drugs (into the hydrophobic compartment of the phospholipid bilayer). For more than 2 decades they have been considered to be promising drug carriers. They are biologically inert and completely biocompatible, and they cause practically no toxic or antigenic reactions; drugs included in liposomes are protected from the destructive action of external media.

Table 1. Some Examples of Liposomal Drugs Approved for Clinical Application or Undergoing Clinical Evaluation for Cancer Therapy

Active Drug (and product name for liposomal preparation)	Indications
Daunorubicin (DaunoXome)	Kaposi's sarcoma
Doxurubicin (Mycet)	Combinational therapy of recurrent breast cancer
Doxorubicin in polyethylene glycol liposomes (Doxil, Caelyx)	Refractory Kaposi's sarcoma; ovarian cancer; recurrent breast cancer
Vincristine (Onco TCS)	Non-Hodgkin's lymphoma
Lurtotecan (NX211)	Ovarian cancer
All-trans retinoic acid (Altragen)	Acute promyelocytic leukemia; non-Hodgkin's lymphoma; renal cell carcinoma; Kaposi's sarcoma
Platinum compounds (Platar)	Solid tumors
Annamycin	Doxorubicin-resistant tumors
DNA plasmid encoding HLA-B7 and β2 microglobulin (Allovectin-7)	Metastatic melanoma
Liposomes for various drugs and diagnostic agents (LipoMASC)	Various applications

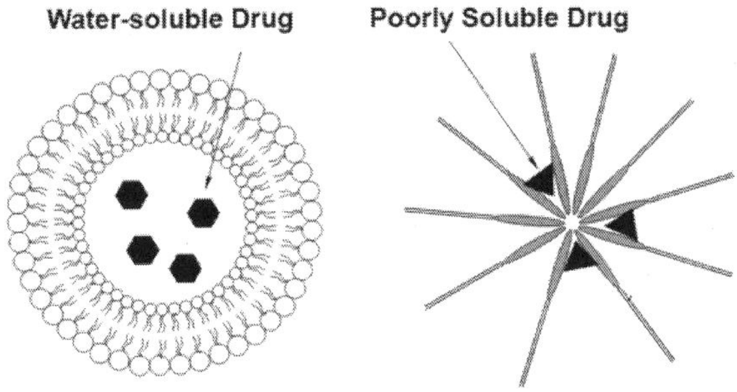

Figure : Schematic pictures of the liposome (left) and micelle (right) and their load with various drugs.

The use of targeted liposomes, that is, liposomes selectively accumulating inside an affected organ or tissue, increases the efficacy of the liposomal drug and decreases the loss of liposomes and their contents in the reticuloendothelial system (RES). To obtain targeted liposomes, many protocols have been developed to bind corresponding targeting moieties, including antibodies, to the liposome surface without affecting the liposome integrity and antibody properties. However, the approach with immunoliposomes may nevertheless be limited because of their short life in the circulation.

Dramatically better accumulation can be achieved if the circulation time of liposomes is extended, increasing the total quantity of immunoliposomes passing through the target and increasing their interactions with target antigens. This is why long-circulated (usually, coated with PEG, ie, PEGylated) liposomes have attracted so much attention over the last decade. It was demonstrated that the unique properties of long-circulating and targeted liposomes could be combined in 1 preparation in which antibodies or other specific binding molecules had been attached to the water-exposed tips of PEG chains.

The development of drug nanocarriers for poorly soluble pharmaceuticals is an important task, particularly because large proportions of new drug candidates emerging from high-throughput drug screening initiatives are water-insoluble, but there are some unresolved issues.

The therapeutic application of hydrophobic, poorly water-soluble agents is associated with some serious problems, since low water-solubility results in poor absorption and low bioavailability. In addition, drug aggregation upon intravenous administration of poorly soluble drugs might lead to such complications as embolism and local toxicity. On the other hand, the hydrophobicity and low solubility in water appear to be intrinsic properties of many drugs, since it helps a drug molecule to penetrate a cell membrane and reach important intracellular targets. To overcome the poor solubility of certain drugs, the use of various micelle-forming surfactants in formulations of insoluble drugs is suggested. This is why micelles, including polymeric micelles, are another promising type of pharmaceutical carrier. Micelles are colloidal dispersions with a particle size between 5 nm and 100 nm.

An important property of micelles is their ability to increase the solubility and bioavailability of poorly soluble pharmaceuticals. The use of certain special amphiphilic molecules as micelle building blocks can also extend the blood half-life upon intravenous administration. Because of their small size (5-100 nm), micelles demonstrate spontaneous penetration into the interstitium in the body compartments with leaky vasculature (tumors and infarcts) by the EPR effect-a form of selective delivery termed "passive targeting." It has been repeatedly shown that micelle-incorporated anticancer drugs, such as adriamycin accumulate better in tumors than in nontarget tissues, thus minimizing undesired drug toxicity toward normal tissue. Diffusion and accumulation parameters for drug carriers in tumors have recently been shown to be strongly dependent on the cutoff size of the tumor blood vessel wall, and the cutoff size varies for different tumors.

Specific ligands (e.g, antibodies and/or certain sugar moieties) can be attached to the water-exposed termini of hydrophilic blocks. In the case of targeted micelles, local release of a free drug from micelles in the target organ should lead to increased efficacy of the drug, while the stability of the micelles en route to the target organ or tissue should contribute better drug solubility and toxicity reduction, because of less interaction with nontarget organs.

By virtue of their small size and by functionalizing their surface with synthetic polymers and appropriate ligands, nanoparticulate carriers can be targeted to specific cells and locations within the body after intravenous or subcutaneous injection. Such approaches may enhance detection sensitivity in medical imaging, improve therapeutic effectiveness, and decrease side effects. Some of the carriers can be engineered in such a way that they can be activated by changes in the environmental pH, by chemical stimuli, by the application of a rapidly oscillating magnetic field, or by application of an external heat source.

Such modifications offer control over particle integrity, drug delivery rates, and the location of drug release, for example, within specific organelles. Some carriers are being designed with a focus on multifunctionality, targeting cell receptors and delivering drugs and biological sensors simultaneously. Some include the incorporation of 1 or more nanosystems within other carriers, as in micellar encapsulation of quantum dots; this allows to follow their inherent nonspecific adsorption and aggregation in biological environments.

THE DRUG DELIVERY FOR CANCER TREATMENT

Core features of cancer cell

- Abnormal growth control
- Improved cell survival
- Abnormal differentiation
- Unlimited replicated potential
- Host-tumor symbiosis

Transport of an anticancer drug in interestium will be governed by physiological (i.e. pressure) and physiochemical (i.e. composition, structure and charge) properties of the interestium and by the physiochemical properties of molecules (size, configuration, charge and hydrophobicity) itself. Thus, to deliver therapeutic agents to tumor cells in vivo, one must overcome the following problems:

- Drug resistance at the tumor level due to physiological barriers (non cellular based mechanisms),
- Drug resistance at the cellular level (cellular mechanisms),
- Distribution, biotransformation and clearance of anticancer drugs in the body.

A strategy could be to associate antitumor drugs with colloidal nanoparticles, with the aim to overcome non-cellular and cellular based mechanisms of resistance and to increase selectivity of drugs towards cancer cells while reducing their toxicity towards normal tissues. There are different drug delivery strategies that have been used to fight with cancer which are discussed in this paper.

Drug Delivery Strategies used to Fight Cancers

There are a variety of different delivery strategies that are either currently being used or are in the testing stage to treat human cancers which are discussed in this paper.

Variety of different drug delivery strategies

Direct Introduction of anticancer drugs into tumor

- Injection Directly into the tumor
- Tumor necrosis therapy
- Injection into the arterial blood supply of cancer
- Local injection into the tumor for radiopotentiation

- Localized delivery of anticancer drugs by electroporation (Electrochemotherapy)
- Local delivery by anticancer drugs implants

Routes of Drug delivery

- Intraperitoneal
- Intrathecal
- Nasal
- Oral
- Pulmonary inhalation
- Subcutaneous injection or implant
- Transdermal drug delivery
- Vascular route: intravenous, intra-arterial

Systematic delivery targeted to tumor

- Heat-activated targeted drug delivery
- Tissue-selective drug delivery for cancer using carrier-mediated transport systems
- Tumor-activated produrg therapy for targeted delivery of chemotherapy
- Pressure-induced filtration of drug across vessels to tumor
- Promoting selective permeation of the anticancer agent into the tumor
- Two-step targeting using bispecific antibody
- Site-specific delivery and light-activation of anticancer proteins

Drug delivery targeted to blood vessels of tumor

- Antiangiogenesis therapy
- Angiolytic therapy
- Drugs to induce clotting in blood vessels of tumor
- Vascular targeting agents

Special formulations and carriers of anticancer drugs

- Albumin based drug carriers
- Carbohydrate-enhanced chemotherapy
- Delivery of proteins and peptides for cancer therapy
- Fatty acids as targeting vectors linked to active drugs
- Microspheres
- Monoclonal antibodies

- Nanoparticles
- Pegylated liposomes (enclosed in a polyethylene glycol bilayer)
- Polyethylene glycol (PEG) technology
- Single-chain antigen-binding technology

Transmembrane drug delivery to intracellular targets

- Cytoporter
- Receptor-mediated endocytosis
- Transduction of proteins and Peptides
- Vitamins as carriers for anticancer agents

Biological Therapies

- Antisense therapy
- Cell therapy
- Gene therapy
- Genetically modified bacteria
- Oncolytic viruses
- RNA interference

Nanoparticle Pathways in Cancer Drug Delivery

Nanotechnology has tremendous potential to make an important contribution in cancer prevention, detection, diagnosis, imaging and treatment. It can target a tumor, carry imaging capability to document the presence of tumor, sense pathophysiological defects in tumor cells, deliver therapeutic genes or drugs based on tumor characteristics, respond to external triggers to release the agent and document the tumor response and identify residual tumor cells.

Nanoparticles are important because of their nanoscaled structure but nanoparticles in cancer are still bigger than many anticancer drugs.

Their "large" size can make it difficult for them to evade organs such as the liver, spleen, and lungs, which are constantly clearing foreign materials from the body. In addition, they must be able to take advantage of subtle differences in cells to distinguish between normal and cancerous tissues. Indeed, it is only recently that researchers have begun to successfully engineer nanoparticles that can effectively evade the immune system and actively target tumors. Active tumor targeting of nanoparticles involves attaching molecules, known collectively as ligands to the outsides of nanoparticles.

These ligands are special in that they can recognize and bind to complementary molecules, or receptors, found on the surface of tumor cells. When such targeting molecules are added to a drug delivery nanoparticle, more of the anticancer drug finds and enters the tumor cell, increasing the efficacy of the treatment and reducing toxic effects on surrounding normal tissues.

Although the past 30 years of innovation in nanotechnology has removed much of the "magic" to yield 21st century "smart bombs" capable of carrying a whole host of new anticancer drugs directly to tumors, we are still searching for the ideal delivery nanosystem. Nanotechnology studies are not new. In essence, all drug molecules can be considered as Nanoengineered structures. What is new is the inclusion of a number of other nano-based approaches to medical studies.

TARGETING THROUGH STIMULI SENSITIVITY

The development of stimuli-sensitive nanocarriers is a hot issue in nanomedicine for cancer. The concept is based on the fact that tumors normally have a lower pH value and a higher temperature than normal tissue, and stimuli-sensitive nanocarriers can be built releasing the incorporated drug only when subjected to these "special" conditions of the tumor.

One has to realize that the stability of PEGylated nanocarriers may not always be favorable for drug delivery to and into tumor cells.

In particular, if drug-containing nanocarriers accumulate inside the tumor, they may be unable to release the drug easily to kill the tumor cells. Likewise, if the carrier has to be taken up by a cell via an endocytic pathway, the presence of the PEG coat on its surface may preclude the contents from escaping the endosome and being delivered into the cytoplasm.

To solve these problems, for example, in the case of long-circulating liposomes, the chemistry was developed to detach PEG from the lipid anchor in the desired conditions.

Labile linkage that would degrade only in the acidic conditions characteristic of the endocytic vacuole or the acidotic tumor mass can be based on the diortho esters,132 vinyl esters,133 cysteine-cleavable lipopolymers, double esters, and hydrazones that are quite stable at pH around 7.5 but are hydrolyzed relatively fast at pH values of 6 and below.

Polymeric components with pH-sensitive (pH-cleavable) bonds are used to produce stimuli-responsive drug delivery systems that are stable in the circulation or in normal tissues but acquire the ability to degrade and release the entrapped drugs in body areas or cell compartments with lowered pH, such as tumors, or cell cytoplasm or endosomes.

A variety of liposomes and polymeric micelles have been described that include the components with acid-labile bonds.

Serum-stable, long-circulating PEGylated pH-sensitive liposomes were also prepared using the combination of PEG and the pH-sensitive terminally alkylated copolymer of N-isopropylacrylamide and methacrylic on the same liposome, since the attachment of the pH-sensitive polymer to the surface of liposomes might facilitate liposome destabilization and drug release in compartments with decreased pH values.

The combination of pH sensitivity and specific ligand targeting for cytosolic drug delivery using decreased endosomal pH values was described for folate- and Tf-targeted liposomes.

Mixed micelle made of pH-sensitive components (polyhistidine and polylactic acid) loaded with adriamycin and targeted to tumors with folate residue provided better drug release under lowered pH values and demonstrated better killing of MCF-7 cells in vitro.

Such micelles can be prepared from different components and loaded with different drugs, and they have already demonstrated their utility in vivo. They have also been shown to suppress even drug-resistant tumor cells effectively. Similar data have been also obtained with temperature-sensitive micelles.

The stimuli sensitivity of PEG coats can also allow for the preparation of multifunctional drug delivery systems with temporarily "hidden" functions, which under normal circumstances are "shielded" by the protective PEG coat but become exposed after PEG detaches.

A nanoparticular drug delivery system can be prepared so that it accumulates in the required organ or tissue and then penetrates inside target cells, delivering its load (drug or DNA) there. The initial target (tumor, infarct) accumulation could be achieved by passive targeting via the EPR effect or by specific ligand (antibody)-mediated active targeting, whereas the subsequent intracellular delivery could be mediated by certain internalizable ligands (folate, transferrin) or by cell-penetrating peptides (CPPs, e.g, TAT or polyArg).

When in the blood, the cell-penetrating function should be temporarily inactivated (sterically shielded) to prevent nonspecific drug delivery into nontarget cells. However, when inside the target, the nanocarrier loses its protective coat, exposes the cell-penetrating function, and provides intracellular drug delivery. Systems like this one require that multiple functions attached to the surface of the nanocarrier work in a certain orchestrated and coordinated way. For the above system the following requirements have to be met:

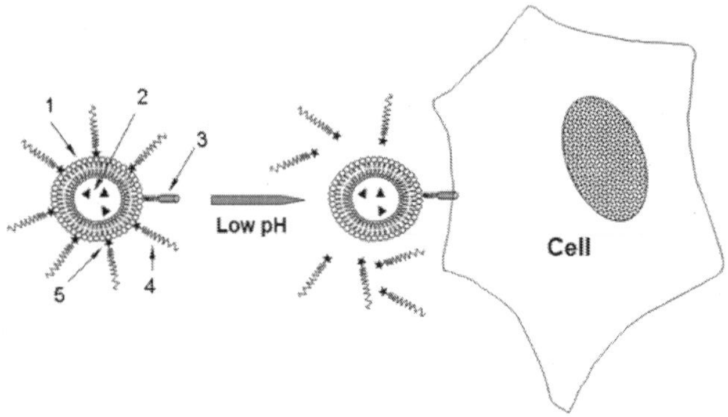

Figure : Targeting with the "hidden" function. The nanocarrier (1) is loaded with the drugs (2) and modified with the cell-penetrating function (3). Additionally, the nanocarrier is coated with a sterically protecting polymer (4) attached to the surface with the pH-sensitive bond (5). When in the blood, the cell-penetrating function is sterically shielded by the protective polymer chains, and the carrier accumulates in the tumor via the enhanced permeability and retention effect. Inside the tumor, local low pH causes the detachment of the protective polymer and the exposure of the cell-penetrating function, which then brings the carrier and the drug inside the tumor cells.

(1) the life of the carrier in the circulation should be long enough to fit EPR effect or targeted delivery requirements (ie, the PEG coat mediating the longevity function or the specific ligand mediating the targeting function should not be lost by the nanocarrier when in the circulation), and (2) the internalization of the carrier within the target cells should proceed sufficiently fast so as not to allow for carrier degradation and drug loss in the interstitial space (i.e, local stimuli-dependent removal of the protective function and the exposure of the temporarily hidden second function should proceed fast).

Targeting Tumors for Diagnostic Visualization

Whatever imaging modality (gamma-scintigraphy, MR imaging, or computed tomography) is used, medical diagnostic imaging requires that sufficient intensity of a corresponding signal from an area of interest be achieved in order to differentiate this area from the surrounding tissues. Unfortunately, nonenhanced imaging techniques are useful only when relatively large tissue areas are involved in the pathological process. To solve the problem and to achieve a sufficient attenuation in the case of small lesions, contrast agents are used that are able to absorb certain types of signal (irradiation) much stronger than surrounding tissues. The contrast agents are specific for each imaging modality, and as a result of their accumulation in certain sites of interest, those sites may be easily visualized when the appropriate imaging modality is applied.

To further increase local spatial concentration of a contrast agent for better imaging, it was suggested that clinicians use certain nanoparticulate carriers able to carry multiple contrast moieties for efficient delivery of contrast agents to areas of interest and enhancement of signals from these areas. Among nanocarriers for contrast agents, liposomes and micelles have received special attention because of their easily controlled properties and good pharmacological characteristics. Liposomes may incorporate contrast agents in both the internal aqueous compartment and the membrane. Two general approaches are used to prepare liposomes for gamma and MR imaging. First, the reporter metal is chelated into a soluble chelate (e.g, diethylenetriamine pentaacetate [DTPA]) and then included in the interior of a liposome.

Alternatively, DTPA or a similar chelating compound may be chemically derivatized by the incorporation of a hydrophobic group, which can anchor the chelating moiety onto the liposome surface during or after liposome preparation. Different chelators and different hydrophobic anchors were tried for the preparation of 111 In, 99mTc, Mn-, and Gd-liposomes. In the case of MR imaging, for a better MR signal, all reporter atoms should be freely exposed for interaction with water. Membranotropic chelating agents-such as DTPA-stearylamine (DTPA-SA) or DTPA-phosphatidyl ethanolamine (DTPA-PE)-consist of the polar head containing a chelated paramagnetic atom, and the lipid moiety that anchors the metal-chelate complex in the liposome membrane. Liposomes with membrane-bound paramagnetic ion demonstrate also a reduced risk of leakage of potentially toxic metals in the body.

The amphiphilic chelating probes (paramagnetic Gd-DTPA-PE and radioactive 111In-DTPA-SA) were also incorporated into PEG(5 kDa)-PE micelles and used in vivo for MR and scintigraphy imaging. In micelles, the lipid part of the molecule can be anchored in the micelle's hydrophobic core while a more hydrophilic chelate is localized on the hydrophilic shell of the micelle. The main feature that makes PEG-lipid micelles attractive for diagnostic imaging applications is their small size, which allows for good intratumoral accumulation of diagnostic micelles.

To further increase liposome load with diagnostic moieties, polychelating amphiphilic polymers (PAP) were synthesized consisting of the main chain with multiple side chelating groups capable of firm binding many reporter metal atoms and a hydrophobic terminal group, allowing for polymer adsorption onto hydrophobic nanoparticles or incorporation into hydrophobic domains of liposomes or micelles. Such surface modification of nanocarriers allows for a sharp increase in the number of bound reporter metal atoms per particle and the image signal intensity. In the case of MR, metal atoms chelated into polymer side groups are directly exposed to the water environment, which enhances the relaxivity of the paramagnetic ions and leads to a corresponding enhancement of the vesicle contrast properties.

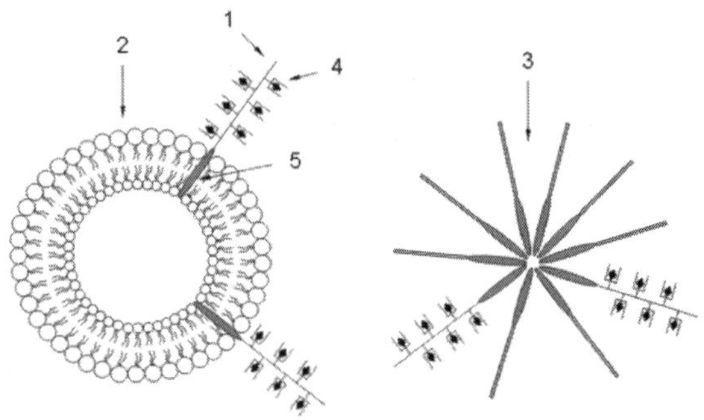

Figure : The incorporation of the amphiphilic polychelating polymer (1) into the liposome membrane (2) or micelle core (3). Each polychelating chain contains multiple chelating groups (4), which carry diagnostic heavy-metal atoms (eg, 111In or 99mTc for gamma-scintigraphy or Gd or Mn for magnetic resonance imaging) and a hydrophobic tail (5) to anchor the liposome or micelle.

An interesting example of the application of PAP-nanoparticles in vivo is the MR imaging of lymphatic system components with Gd-loaded nanocarriers (important for discovering metastases in lymph nodes). Liposomes and micelles have been studied as delivery vehicles to the lymphatic system. It has been shown that radioactively labeled small negatively charged liposomes are the most efficient in targeting rat regional lymph nodes after subcutaneous administration. The optimal diameter of liposomes that localize in the lymph nodes after peritoneal administration in rats is ~200 nm. Liposomes loaded with chelated paramagnetic ions (mostly Gd, Dy, Mn, Fe) have been demonstrated to be useful as MR imaging contrast agents, mostly for the visualization of macrophage-rich tissues, such as the organs of the RES.

In experimental rabbits, transverse scans obtained after subcutaneous administration of a suspension of Gd-PAP-liposomes into the right forepaw demonstrated that axillary and subscapular lymph nodes can be seen on a scan taken only 5 minutes postinjection. The approach was additionally proved by fast and informative diagnostic visualization of VX_2 human sarcoma in rabbit popliteal lymph node, when with 200 nm of Gd-PAP-liposomes a tumor was clearly seen 10 minutes postinjection. The overall performance of Gd-PAP-liposomes or-micelles in lymph node visualization might be further improved by additional incorporation of amphiphilic PEG onto the liposome membrane or micelle surface, which can be explained by increased $1/T_1$ values of PEG-Gd-liposomes due to the presence of an increased amount of PEG-associated water protons in the close vicinity of chelated Gd ions located on the liposomal membrane. In addition to the enhanced relaxivity, the coating of the liposome surface with PEG polymer can help in avoiding contrast agent uptake in the site of injection by resident phagocytic cells.

The ability of various PEG-liposomal formulations labeled with ^{67}Ga, ^{111}In, or ^{99m}Tc to localize in tumors has been demonstrated in a series of preclinical studies. In fact, numerous successful tumor detection studies were done with contrast-loaded long-circulating liposomes using human tumor xenografts in nude mice. Moreover, the clinical data on 111In-labeled long-circulating liposomes are already available on the visualization of lung cancer, head and neck cancers, AIDS-related Kaposi's sarcoma, skin cancer, glioblastomas and metastatic brain tumors, soft tissue sarcomas, and other malignancies.

^{111}In-DTPA-labeled PEGylated liposomes (prepared using the ^{111}In-oxine method) have also been used to study the biodistribution and the pharmacokinetics of long-circulating liposomes and to assess their applicability for the radioimaging of tumor localization and evaluation of different therapeutic treatment strategies against various types of cancers. Clinically, successful tumor imaging was achieved in 15 of 17 patients with cancer (4 of 5 breast, 5 of 5 head and neck, 3 of 4 bronchus, 2 of 2 glioma, and 1 of 1 cervix).

Koukourakis et al investigated the accumulation of ^{99m}Tc-DTPA-radiolabeled long-circulating liposomal doxorubicin (Doxil) in 10 patients with metastatic brain tumors and five patients with brain glioblastoma undergoing radiotherapy. Radiolabeled Doxil accumulation was 13 to 19 times higher in the glioblastomas and 7 to 13 times higher in the metastatic lesions, as compared with the normal brain. Belhaj-Tayeb et al have recently suggested an original method to encapsulate ^{99m}Tc-MIBI in preformed PEG liposomes. They used an exchange with an efflux of K+ through the valinomycin ionophores, that is, an active encapsulation, which resulted in 50% encapsulation efficiency of 99mTc-MIBI in PEG liposomes. One hour postinjection in rats, PEG liposomes showed a 10 times higher activity in blood than free ^{99m}Tc-MIBI, whereas the activity of free 99mTc-MIBI in kidneys and bladder was markedly higher than that of encapsulated ^{99m}Tc-MIBI, indicating faster clearance of the free radiotracer. In the breast cancer (MCF7-ras)-bearing nude mice, PEG liposome uptake in tumors was 2 times that for the free ^{99m}Tc-MIBI. Overall, the ^{99m}Tc-MIBI-PEG liposomes demonstrated not only longer blood circulation time but also improved tumor-to-background ratio in the in vivo imaging.

Based on the fact that vasoactive intestinal peptide receptors (VIP-R) are approximately 5 times more expressed in human breast cancer compared with normal breast tissue, Dagar et al125 used VIP, a 28-amino-acid mammalian neuropeptide, as a breast cancer targeting moiety for targeted imaging of breast cancer. VIP was covalently attached to the surface of long-circulating liposomes that encapsulated the ^{99m}Tc-HMPAO complex. It was found that the presence of VIP did not affect the size and ^{99m}Tc-HMPAO encapsulation ability of the liposomes and did not alter the pharmacokinetic profile of the PEGylated liposomal formulation. Liposomes with and without VIP on their surface accumulated at significantly higher quantities in breast cancer when compared with normal breast in rats, indicating the EPR-dependent passive targeting of these formulations to cancer tissues. Still, in breast cancer, ^{99m}Tc-HMPAO liposomes modified with VIP showed significantly more accumulation than did analogs without VIP. The tumor-to-nontumor ratio was also significantly higher for ^{99m}Tc-HMPAO liposomes modified with VIP than for VIP-free ^{99m}Tc-HMPAO liposomes, suggesting active targeting of VIP liposomes to breast cancer.

In general, nanoparticles are believed to be used as modular platforms to build a broad variety of targeted imaging agents, since multiple molecules of imaging agents and cancer-specific ligands can be assembled into a single nanoparticle. Multifunctional magnetic nanocrystals coupled with a cancer-specific antibody, Herceptin, allowed for successful in vivo MR detection of cancer.186 Anticancer antibodies were shown to effectively accumulate contrast agent-loaded pharmaceutical nanocarriers in tumors and provide for faster and better visualization. Simultaneous cancer cell imaging and photodynamic therapy in the near-infrared region can be performed using gold nanorods because of strong adsorption and scattering of electromagnetic radiation by noble-metal nanoparticles. The conjugation of cancer-specific antibody with such nanorods results in the preparation providing selective killing of cancer cells upon the exposure to a red laser at 800 nm. Use of the same principle was suggested for early optical detection of cancer with gold nanoshells.

Miscellaneous Tumor Targeting

Photodynamic therapy (PDT) is a fast-developing modality for the treatment of superficial tumors, where photosensitizing agents are used for photochemical eradication of malignant cells. In PDT, liposomes are used both as drug carriers and as enhancers. Targeting as well as the controlled release of photosensitizing agent in tumors may still further increase the outcome of the liposome-mediated PDT. Benzoporphyrin derivative encapsulated in polycation liposomes modified with cetyl-PEI was used for antiangiogenic PDT. This drug in such liposomes was better internalized by human umbilical vein endothelial cells and was found in the intranuclear region and associated with mitochondria.

Another porphyrin derivative (SIM01) in dimyristoyl phosphatidylcholine liposomes also gives better results in PDT, mainly because of better accumulation in the tumor (human adenocarcinoma in nude mice). Targeting of a poorly soluble PDT agent, meso tetraphenylporphine, solubilized by polymeric micelles modified with a cancer-specific antibody resulted in more efficient killing of cancer cells under the conditions of PDT.

Liposomes are also used for targeting of antisense oligonucleotides, in particular for neuroblastoma treatment, exemplified by coated cationic liposomes made of a central core of a cationic phospholipid bound to oligonucleotide, and an outer shell of neutral lipid. Such liposomes are additionally modified with a monoclonal antibody against neuroectoderma antigen and target antigen-positive cells both in vitro and in vivo.

An interesting approach to the use of targeted liposomes loaded with enzymes in cancer therapy is their application for antibody-directed enzyme prodrug therapy based on the on-site activation of chemically modified inactive phospholipid derivatives of various anticancer and antiviral agents. The application of phospholipid prodrugs incorporated into liposome membranes brings several benefits: the efficiency of the prodrug incorporation is high; prodrugs do not leak from the liposome into the aqueous phase; drugs are protected against metabolic degradation; and long-lasting therapeutic drug levels can be achieved. For specific generation of active cytotoxic molecules from inactive prodrugs in the vicinity of tumor cells, a conjugate of a tumor-specific antibody with an enzyme responsible for the conversion of a prodrug into the active drug is targeted toward the tumor. To increase the efficiency of the required enzyme in the tumor, rather than just "straight" antibody-enzyme conjugates, immunoliposomes were loaded with the required enzyme (immunoenzymosomes).

An emerging area in cancer nanomedicine is now associated with the use of magnetic nanoparticles for different purposes. Thus, the suspensions of coated superparamagnetic nanoparticles were shown to be taken up by cancer cells and can kill those cancer cells after being subjected to an alternating current (AC) magnetic field because of developing hyperthermia. The procedure is termed "magnetic thermal ablation" and has proved itself in various models, including breast cancer models. A similar approach reduced tumor growth in the orthotopic model of prostate cancer in rats.

Moreover, the first clinical results from the use of magnetic nanoparticles for AC-mediated hyperthermia are quite encouraging. This treatment can also be successfully combined with external radiation therapy, as was shown in the rat model. It is especially important that this technique is applicable even to brain tumors, as was shown in rats with malignant glioma. To further enhance the efficacy of this therapy, magnetic particles have been coupled with antitumor antibodies to provide better localization in the tumor, as was shown in an experiment with magnetic nanoparticles targeted to tumors, then subjected to hyperthermia with an external alternating magnetic field.

Intracellular Delivery of Drugs and DNA

Intracellular transport of biologically active molecules with therapeutic properties is one of the key problems in drug delivery. Many pharmaceutical agents need to be delivered intracellularly to exert their therapeutic action inside cytoplasm or onto individual cell organelles. Thus, intracellular drug delivery can overcome certain important limitations for drug action, such as multidrug resistance in cancer chemotherapy. However, the very nature of cell membranes prevents proteins, peptides, and nanoparticulate drug carriers from entering cells unless there is an active transport mechanism, which is usually the case for very short peptides.204 So far, multiple and only partially successful attempts have been made to bring various low-molecular-weight and macromolecular drugs and drug-loaded pharmaceutical carriers directly into the cell cytoplasm, bypassing the endocytic pathway, to protect drugs and DNA from lysosomal degradation, thus enhancing drug efficiency or DNA incorporation into the cell genome.

However, even being safely delivered into the cell cytoplasm, drugs still have to find their way to specific organelles (nuclei, mitochondria), where they are expected to use their therapeutic potential. Various vector molecules promote the delivery of associated drugs and drug carriers inside the cells via receptor-mediated endocytosis. This process involves attachment of the vector molecule and an associated drug carrier to specific ligands on target cell membranes, followed by the energy-dependent formation of endosomes. The problem, however, is that any molecule/particle entering the cell via the endocytic pathway and becoming trapped in the endosome eventually ends in the lysosome, where active degradation processes take place under the action of lysosomal enzymes. As a result, only a small fraction of unaffected substance appears in the cell cytoplasm. Thus, even if efficient cellular uptake via endocytosis is observed, the delivery of intact peptides and proteins is compromised by insufficient endosomal escape and subsequent lysosomal degradation.

pH-Sensitive Carriers

Quite a few approaches for cytosolic drug delivery with such pharmaceutical nanocarriers as liposomes and micelles have been developed. Among the different methods of liposomal content delivery into the cytoplasm it was proposed that the liposome is made of pH-sensitive components and, after being endocytosed in the intact form, it fuses with the endovacuolar membrane under the action of lowered pH inside the endosome (below 6) and destabilizes the endosome, releasing its content directly into the cytoplasm. Thus, endosomes become the gates from the outside into the cell cytoplasm.

Cellular drug delivery mediated by pH-sensitive liposomes is not a simple intracellular leakage from the lipid vesicle since the drug has to cross the endosomal membrane as well. It is usually assumed that inside the endosome, the low pH and some other factors destabilize the liposomal membrane, which, in turn, interacts with the endosomal membrane, provoking its secondary destabilization and drug release into the cytoplasm. The presence of fusogenic lipids in the liposome composition, such as unsaturated dioleoylphosphatidylethanolamine (DOPE), with their ability to easily adopt an inverted hexagonal phase, is usually required to make liposomes pH-sensitive. Importantly (since many current liposomal dosage forms are based on the use of long-circulating, PEGylated liposomes), long-circulating PEGylated DOPE-containing liposomes, although demonstrating decreased pH sensitivity compared with non-PEGylated liposomes, still effectively delivered their contents into the cytoplasm.

The combination of liposome pH sensitivity and specific ligand targeting for cytosolic drug delivery using decreased endosomal pH values was described for both folate and Tf-targeted liposomes. Additional modification of pH-sensitive liposomes with an antibody results in pH-sensitive immunoliposomes. The advantages of antibody-bearing pH-sensitive liposome include cytoplasmic delivery, targetability, and facilitated uptake (i.e, improved intracellular availability) via receptor-mediated endocytosis. Successful application of pH-sensitive immunoliposomes has been demonstrated in delivery of a variety of molecules, including antitumor drugs.

In addition to membrane-destabilizing lipid components, there exist a large number of membrane-destabilizing anionic polymers that also can enhance the endosomal escape of various drugs and biomacromolecules. This family includes various carboxylated polymers, copolymers of acrylic and methacrylic acids, copolymers of maleic acid, and polymers and copolymers of N-isopropylacrylamide (NIPAM). Copolymers of NIPAM demonstrate a lower critical solution (solubility/insolubility switch) at physiological temperatures and when precipitated, destabilize biomembranes with which they interact. Such polymers can be attached to the surface of drug-/DNA-loaded liposomes or polymeric micelles, allowing for endosomal destabilization and cytoplasmic escape.

Since micelle-based preparations of various poorly water-soluble drugs are considered to be promising dosage forms for such drugs, and since many of those drugs (e.g, paclitaxel) target intracellular organelles, various micelles (polymeric micelles) have been prepared that can also demonstrate pH sensitivity and the ability to escape from endosomes.

Thus, micelles prepared from PEG-poly(aspartate hydrazone adriamycin) easily release an active drug at lower pH values typical for endosomes and facilitate its cytoplasmic delivery and toxicity against cancer cells.215 It is also possible to enhance the intracellular delivery of drug-loaded micelles by adding to their composition the lipid components used in membrane-destabilizing Lipofectin.

Thus, PEG-lipid micelles, for example, carry a net negative charge, which might hinder their internalization by cells. On the other hand, it is known that a net positive charge usually enhances the uptake of various nanoparticles by cells, and after endocytosis, the drug-/DNA-loaded particles could escape from the endosomes and enter a cell's cytoplasm through disruptive interaction of the cationic lipid with endosomal membranes. The compensation for the micelle negative charge by the addition of positively charged lipids to PEG-PE micelles could improve the uptake by cancer cells of drug-loaded mixed PEG-PE/positively charged lipid micelles.

It is also possible that after the enhanced endocytosis, such micelles could escape from the endosomes and enter the cytoplasm of cancer cells. With this in mind, an attempt was made to increase the intracellular delivery and thus the anticancer activity of the micellar paclitaxel by preparing paclitaxel-containing micelles from the mixture of PEG-PE and Lipofectin lipids (LL).

When the cellular uptake of various fluorescently labeled micelles in adherent BT-20 cells was studied, it was found that while both "plain" PEG-PE micelles and PEG-PE/LL micelles were endocytosed by BT-20 cells, as confirmed by the presence of fluorescent endosomes in cells after 2 hours of co-incubation with fluorescently labeled micelles, in case of PEG-PE/LL micelles, endosomes became partially disrupted and their content was released into the cell cytosol.

The addition of LL, facilitating the intracellular uptake and cytoplasmic release of paclitaxel-containing PEG-PE/LL micelles, resulted in a substantially increased level of cell death compared with that under the action of free paclitaxel or paclitaxel delivered using noncationic LL-free PEG-PE micelles. In BT-20 cancer cells, the IC50 values of free paclitaxel, paclitaxel in PEG-PE micelles, and paclitaxel in PEG-PE/LL micelles were 24.3, 9.5, and 6.4 μM, respectively. In A2780 cancer cells, the IC50 values for the same preparations were 22.5, 5.8, and 1.2 μM, respectively.

Delivery by CPPs

A novel and interesting approach to delivering various drug and DNA molecules and even drug-loaded nanoparticles inside cells for cancer therapy involves their modification with CPPs-proteins and peptides that can facilitate uptake through the cellular membranes-thereby enhancing the delivery of CPP-modified molecules inside the cell.

During the last decade, several proteins and peptides have been found to traverse through the cellular membranes, delivering their cargo molecules into the cytoplasm and/or nucleus. Thus, 86-mer transactivating transcriptional activator (TAT) from HIV-1 was efficiently taken up by various cells, when added to the surrounding media.

Subsequently, this property of translocation was found in Antennapedia (Antp), a transcription factor of Drosophila,220 and VP22, a herpes virus protein. Their ability to translocate across the plasma membranes is confined to short sequences within these proteins of fewer than 20 amino acids, which are highly rich in basic residues.

These peptides have been used for intracellular delivery of various cargoes with molecular weights several times greater than their own. Cellular delivery using CPPs has several advantages over conventional techniques because it is efficient for a range of cell types and has a potential therapeutic application.

Collectively, the recent data assume more than 1 mechanism for CPP-mediated intracellular delivery of various molecules and particles. CPP-mediated intracellular delivery of large molecules and nanoparticles proceeds via the energy-dependent macropinocytosis, with subsequent enhanced escape from endosome into the cell cytoplasm, while individual CPPs or CPP-conjugated small molecules penetrate cells via electrostatic interactions and hydrogen bonding and do not seem to depend on energy. Direct contact between the translocating moiety and cell membrane or cell membrane-interacting proteoglycans is required for successful intracellular delivery.

Since traversal through cellular membranes represents a major barrier for efficient delivery of macromolecules inside cells, CPPs may ferry various molecules into mammalian cells in vitro and in vivo.

The use of peptides and protein domains with amphipathic sequences for drug and gene delivery across cellular membranes is getting increasing attention. Covalent hitching of proteins, drugs, DNA, or other macromolecules onto CPPs may circumvent conventional limitations by allowing for transport of these compounds into a wide variety of cells in vitro and in vivo.

Herpes simplex virus VP22 protein was used to deliver E2 protein into target cells. Overexpression of the E2 protein in cervical cancer cells can induce growth arrest and/or apoptotic cell death; thus, E2 might be useful in the treatment of cervical cancer. VP22-E2 fusion proteins induced apoptosis in transiently transfected human papillomavirus (HPV)-transformed cervical carcinoma cell lines. When COS-7 cells producing VP22-E2 were seeded into cultures of HPV-transformed cells, VP22-E2 entered the nonproducing cells and induced apoptosis. This suggests that the local delivery of VP22-E2 fusion proteins could be used to treat cervical cancer and other HPV-associated diseases.

VP22 enhanced intercellular trafficking of thymidine kinase (TK) and amplified the TK/ganciclovir (GCV) killing effect, especially in the lower range of GCV concentrations, offering a new strategy to enhance the effectiveness of suicide gene therapy for the treatment of cancers. Chimeric polypeptides of VP22 linked to the entire p53 protein were shown to spread between cells and accumulate in recipient cell nuclei. Also, the VP22-p53 chimeric protein efficiently induced apoptosis in p53 negative human osteosarcoma cells, resulting in a widespread cytotoxic effect.

VP22 was also used to deliver oligonucleotides in vitro and in vivo. Complexes of VP22 with fluorescein-labeled oligonucleotides, termed "vectosomes," were efficiently taken up by cells and remained stable in the cell cytoplasm without any particular activity. These vectosomes were disrupted by light to release the antisense activity. Anti-c-Raf1 vectosomes were efficiently activated by light in vivo after injection into subcutaneous tumors implanted in nude mice and slowed down the tumor growth because of the strong inhibition of c-Raf1 protein expression, the antitumor activity being much higher than that of the antisense alone or of the different control vectosomes.

Suicide gene therapy is a widely exploited approach for gene therapy of cancer and other hyperproliferative disorders. However, it is hampered by the relative inefficiency of TK gene transfer and its limited bystander effect. Fusion of TK to TAT protein transduction domain (PTD) imparted cell membrane translocating ability to the enzyme and significantly increased its cytotoxic efficacy.

The enzyme was present extracellularly in the cells expressing TAT11-TK, associated with the cell surface heparan sulfate proteoglycans, and was released into the cell culture medium. The protein was then internalized by neighboring nonexpressing cells, which underwent apoptosis when treated with the nucleoside analog acyclovir. Thus, development of this approach was an important step in the establishment of TK suicide gene therapy.

The attachment of TATp to a water-soluble synthetic macromolecule, N-(2-hydroxypropyl)methacrylamide copolymer, resulted in the cytoplasmic and nuclear delivery of the conjugate via nonendocytotic and concentration-independent processes, as opposed to conjugates without TATp, which accumulated in only endocytotic vesicles.

Furthermore, the TATp-polymer-bound anticancer drug doxorubicin was delivered inside the cytoplasm, providing the possibility for the development of polymer-based systems for the cytoplasmic delivery of therapeutic molecules.

Another growing application of transduction technology is in the field of cancer therapy, where the transduction methodology appears to circumvent the problems encountered with the conventional chemotherapeutic regimens, such as nonspecificity and exclusion of drugs by efflux transporters in multidrug-resistant cells.

The transduction domains of Antennapedia and TAT have been linked to the tumor suppressor peptide p53, which enhanced the accumulation of p53 in the tumor cells and activated the apoptotic genes for the selective killing of tumor cells both in vitro and in vivo. The TAT peptide has also been used to deliver proteins that modulate the cell cycle and arrest tumor growth. Another approach to selectively killing tumor cells is transducing dendritic cells with tumor antigens to generate cytotoxic lymphocytes that eradicate tumors. The TAT transduction domain was used to transduce dendritic cells with ovalbumin, a recombinant model tumor-associated antigen. The transduced dendritic cells generated cytotoxic lymphocytes against tumors. Immunization with transduced dendritic cells imparted an antitumor immunity and inhibited lung metastases in a 3-day tumor model. Some approaches currently used for intracellular delivery.

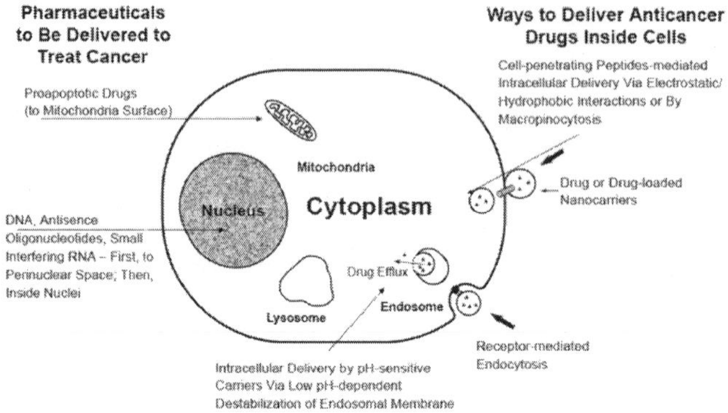

Figure : Schematics of intracellular drug delivery.

SUMMATIVE ANALYSIS

Even a rather brief review of what is going on in the field of tumor-targeted pharmaceutical nanocarriers shows the breadth of this approach. Significant information has accumulated regarding the most convenient carrier systems (e.g, liposomes) and possible ways of using them for the targeted delivery of drugs, imaging agent, and genes into tumors. The most important problem is now associated with the translation of various successfully proven experimental concepts into clinical practice. With evident achievements in the clinical use of some first-generation anticancer nanomedicines (Doxil being a good example), one can expect the appearance of "real" targeted anticancer nanomedicines in the not-too-distant future.

TARGETING CANCER

Role of Nanocarrier Longevity in the Blood

A serious limitation with all pharmaceutical nanocarriers is that the body normally treats them as foreign particles, so they become easily opsonized and removed from the circulation before completion of their function. Thus, one of the most important properties of any pharmaceutical nanocarrier loaded with any anticancer drug is its longevity, and long-circulating pharmaceuticals and pharmaceutical carriers are currently an important and still growing area of biomedical research. There are quite a few important reasons for making long-circulating drugs and drug carriers. One of them is to maintain a required level of a pharmaceutical agent in the blood for extended time intervals. Then, long-circulating drug-containing microparticulates or large macromolecular aggregates can slowly accumulate in pathological sites with affected and leaky vasculature (eg, tumors, inflammations, infarcted areas), and facilitate drug delivery in those areas. In addition, the prolonged circulation can help to achieve a better targeting effect for targeted (specific ligand-modified) drugs and drug carriers, allowing more time for their interaction with the target because of a larger number of passages of targeted pharmaceuticals through the target with the blood.

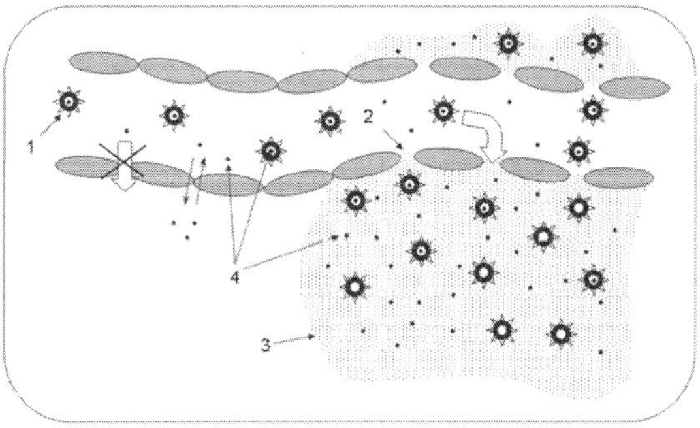

Figure : Enhanced permeability and retention (EPR) effect. Long-circulating drug carriers (1) penetrate through the leaky pathological vasculature (2) into the tumor interstitium (3) and degrade there, releasing a free drug (4) and creating its high local concentration.

Chemical modification of pharmaceutical nanocarriers with certain synthetic polymers, such as PEG, is the approach most frequently used to impart in vivo longevity to drug carriers, as was first suggested for liposomes. Hydrophilic polymers have been shown to protect individual molecules and solid particulates from interaction with different solutes.

The term "steric stabilization" has been introduced to describe the phenomenon of polymer-mediated protection. On the biological level, coating nanoparticles with PEG sterically hinders interactions of blood components with their surface and reduces the binding of plasma proteins with PEGylated nanoparticles, as was demonstrated for liposomes. This approach prevents drug carrier interaction with opsonins and slows down their capture by the RES.

The mechanisms by which PEG prevents opsonization include shielding of the surface charge, increased surface hydrophilicity,56 enhanced repulsive interaction between polymer-coated nanocarriers and blood components, and formation of the polymeric layer over the particle surface, which is impermeable for large molecules of opsonins even at relatively low polymer concentrations. As a protecting polymer, PEG provides a very attractive combination of properties: excellent solubility in aqueous solutions; high flexibility of its polymer chain; very low toxicity, immunogenicity, and antigenicity; lack of accumulation in RES cells; and minimal influence on specific biological properties of modified pharmaceuticals. It is also important that PEG is not biodegradable and subsequently does not form any toxic metabolites. PEG molecules with a molecular weight below 40 kDa are readily excretable from the body via the kidneys. PEG is also easily commercially available in a variety of molecular weights, although PEGs that are normally used for the modification of drug carriers have a molecular weight from 1000 to 20 000 Da. Currently, there are many chemical approaches to synthesizing activated derivatives of PEG and to coupling these derivatives with a variety of drugs and drug carriers.

Pegylated polymeric nanoparticles can also be prepared based on the block-copolymer of PEG and a hydrophobic block, such as polylactide-glycolide (PLAGA). Using PLAGA-PEG copolymer, one can prepare long-circulating particles with an insoluble (solid) PLAGA core and a water-soluble PEG shell covalently linked to the core. Clearance and liver accumulation patterns reveal that the higher the content of PEG blocks, the slower the clearance and the better protection from liver uptake. Similar effects on longevity and biodistribution of microparticular drug carriers might be achieved by direct chemical attachment of protective polyethylene oxide chains onto the surface of preformed particles.

The surface of poly(lactic-glycolic acid) or PLAGA microspheres was also modified by adsorption of the polylysine-PEG copolymer, which resulted in a dramatic decrease of plasma protein adsorption on modified nanoparticles. Similarly, coating polycyanoacrylate particles with PEG resulted in their increased longevity in the circulation, allowing for their diffusion into even the brain tissue. Fluorouracil-containing dendrimer nanoparticles modified with PEG demonstrated better drug retention and less hemolytic activity.

The most significant biological consequence of nanocarrier modification with protecting polymers is a sharp increase in circulation time and decrease in RES (liver) accumulation. This fact is very important clinically, since various long-circulating nanocarriers have been shown to effectively accumulate in many tumors via the EPR effect. Long-circulating liposomes were prepared containing various anticancer agents, such as doxorubicin, arabinofuranosylcytosine, adriamycin, and vincristine. PEG-liposome-incorporated doxorubicin has already demonstrated very good clinical results. From a pharmacokinetic point of view, the association of drugs with any nanocarrier has pronounced effects: delayed drug absorption, restricted drug biodistribution, decreased volume of drug biodistribution, delayed drug clearance, and retarded drug metabolism. The presence of protective polymer on the carrier surface changes all these parameters still further.

Tumor-Targeted Specific Ligands on Long-Circulating Nanocarriers

To achieve better selective targeting by PEG-coated liposomes or other particulates, targeting ligands were attached to nanocarriers via the PEG spacer arm, so that the ligand was extended outside of the dense PEG brush, excluding steric hindrances for its binding to the target receptors. With this in mind, potential ligands were attached to the activated far (distal) ends of some liposome-grafted polymeric chains.27,80 Since PEG-lipid conjugates used for the steric protection of liposomes and other pharmaceutical nanocarriers and for the preparation of polymeric micelles are derived from methoxy-PEG and carry only nonreactive methoxy terminal groups, several attempts have been made to functionalize PEG tips in PEG-lipid conjugates.

For this purpose, several types of end-group functionalized lipopolymers of the general formula X-PEG-PE59, were introduced, where X represents a reactive functional group-containing moiety, while PEG-PE represents the conjugate of polyethylene (PE) and PEG. Most of the end-group functionalized PEG lipids were synthesized from heterobifunctional PEG derivatives containing hydroxyl and carboxyl or amino groups. Typically, the hydroxyl end-group of PEG was derivatized to form a urethane attachment with the hydrophobic lipid anchor, PE, while the amino or carboxyl groups were used for the conjugation reaction or for further functionalization. To further simplify the coupling procedure and to make it applicable for single-step binding of a large variety of amino group-containing ligands (including antibodies, proteins, and small molecules) to the distal end of nanocarrier-attached polymeric chains, amphiphilic PEG derivative, p-nitrophenylcarbonyl-PEG-PE (pNP-PEG-PE), was introduced.

pNP-PEG-PE readily adsorbs on hydrophobic nanoparticles or incorporates into liposomes and micelles via its phospholipid residue, and it easily binds any amino group-containing compound via its water-exposed pNP group, forming a stable and nontoxic urethane (carbamate) bond. The reaction between the pNP group and the ligand amino group proceeds easily and quantitatively at pH around 8.0, while excessive free pNP groups are easily eliminated by spontaneous hydrolysis.

Although various monoclonal antibodies have been shown to deliver liposomes and other nanocarriers to many targets, attempts to optimize the properties of immunoliposomes and long-circulating immunoliposomes continue to be made. The majority of research relates to cancer targeting, which uses a variety of antibodies. Internalizing antibodies are required to achieve significantly improved therapeutic efficacy of antibody-targeted liposomal drugs, as was shown using B-lymphoma cells and internalizable epitopes (CD19) as an example.

An interesting concept was developed to target HER2-overexpressing tumors using anti-HER2 liposomes. In all studied HER2-overexpressing models, immunoliposomes showed potent anticancer activity superior to that of control nontargeted liposomes. In part, this superior activity was attributed to the ability of the immunoliposomes to deliver their load inside the target cells via receptor-mediated endocytosis, which is obviously important if the drug's site of action is located inside the cell. Antibody CC52 against rat colon adenocarcinoma CC531 attached to PEGylated liposomes provided specific accumulation of liposomes in a rat model of metastatic CC531.

We obtained a nice illustration of how the addition of the targeting function onto a long-circulating drug-loaded nanocarrier can significantly enhance the activity of a drug when we demonstrated that the nucleosome-specific monoclonal antibody capable of recognizing various tumor cells via the tumor cell surface-bound nucleosomes improved Doxil targeting to tumor cells and increased its cytotoxicity both in vitro and in vivo.

GD2-targeted immunoliposomes with the novel antitumoral drug fenretinide, which induced apoptosis in neuroblastoma and melanoma cell lines, demonstrated strong antineuroblastoma activity both in vitro and in vivo in mice. scFv antibody-modified liposomes were used to target cytotoxic drugs to biological targets, such as ED-B fibronectin. The combination of immunoliposome and endosome-disruptive peptide improves cytosolic delivery of liposomal drug, increases cytotoxicity, and offers a new approach to constructing targeted liposomal systems, as shown in the case of diphtheria toxin A chain incorporated with the pH-dependent fusogenic peptide diINF-7 into liposomes specific toward ovarian carcinoma.

Surface modification with antibodies was also applied to make some other pharmaceutical nanocarriers cancer-targeted. Nanoparticles made of poly (lactic acid) were surface modified with PEG and with antitransferrin receptor monoclonal antibody to produce PEGylated immunoparticles with a size of ~120 nm that contained about 65 bound antibody molecules per single particle. Mammalian cells (NIH3T3, 32D, Ba/F3, and hybridoma 9E10) were surface modified with distal terminus-activated oleyl-PEG, and various proteins (streptavidin, green fluorescent protein [EGFP], and antibody) were successfully attached to the activated PEG termini. A similar combination of longevity and targetability can also be achieved by using some other specific ligands attached to long-circulating preparations.

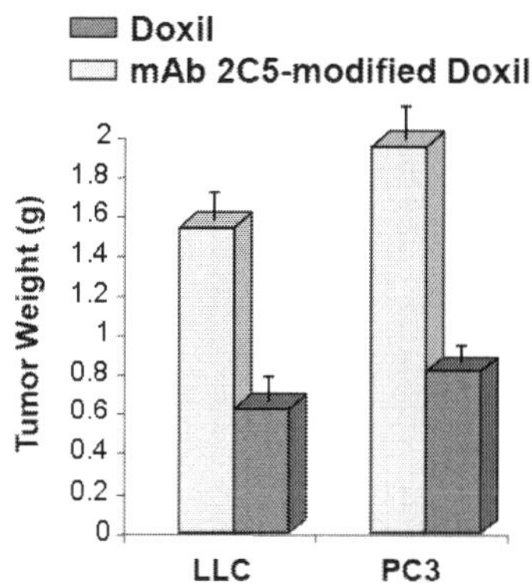

Figure : Antitumor activity in vivo in mice of tumor-specific antibody-modified Doxil compared with unmodified Doxil. LLC indicates Lewis lung carcinoma; PC3, line of prostate carcinoma.

Thus, since transferrin (Tf) receptor (TfR) is overexpressed on the surface of many tumor cells, antibodies against TfR as well as Tf itself are among the ligands popular for targeting various nanoparticular drug carriers, including liposomes, to tumors and inside tumor cells.

Recent studies involve the coupling of Tf to PEG on PEGylated liposomes in order to combine longevity and targetability for drug delivery into solid tumors. A similar approach was applied to deliver into tumors agents for photodynamic therapy, including hypericin, and for intracellular delivery of cisplatin into gastric tumors.

Tf as well as anti-TfR antibodies were also used to facilitate gene delivery into cells by cationic liposomes. Tf-mediated liposome delivery was also successfully used for brain targeting. Immunoliposomes with OX26 monoclonal antibody to the rat TfR were found to concentrate on brain microvascular endothelium.

Targeting tumors with folate-modified nanocarriers is another popular approach, since folate receptor (FR) expression is frequently overexpressed in many tumor cells. Liposomal daunorubicin and doxorubicin were delivered into various tumor cells via folate receptor and demonstrated increased cytotoxicity.

Folate-targeted liposomes have been suggested as delivery vehicles for boron neutron capture therapy and are used also for targeting tumors with haptens for tumor immunotherapy. Folate was also attached to the surface of cyanoacrylate-based nanoparticles via activated PEG blocks. Similarly, PEG-polycaprolactone-based particles were surface-modified with folate and, after being loaded with paclitaxel, demonstrated increased cytotoxicity. Superparamagnetic magnetite nanoparticles were modified with folate (with or without PEG spacer) and demonstrated better uptake by cancer cells, a finding useful for both diagnostic (magnetic resonance [MR] imaging agents) and therapeutic purposes.

As with other delivery systems, the drug delivery potential of polymeric micelles-carriers for poorly soluble anticancer drugs-may also be still further enhanced by attaching targeting ligands to the micelle surface.

The attachment of various specific ligands to the water-exposed termini of hydrophilic blocks could be used to improve the targeting of micelles and micelle-incorporated drugs and DNA. Among those ligands are various sugar moieties, transferrin, and folate residues since many target cells, especially cancer cells, overexpress appropriate receptors (e.g, transferrin and folate receptors) on their surface.

Thus, it was shown that galactose-and lactose-modified micelles made of PEG-polylactide copolymer specifically interact with lectins, thus modeling targeting delivery of the micelles to hepatic sites.

Transferrin-modified micelles based on PEG and poly(ethyleneimine) (PEI) sized between 70 and 100 nm are expected to target tumors with overexpressed transferrin receptors.

Mixed micelle-like complexes of PEGylated DNA and PEI modified with transferring were designed for enhanced DNA delivery into cells overexpressing the same transferrin receptors. A similar targeting approach was successfully tested with folate-modified micelles. Poly(L-histidine)/PEG and poly(L-lactic acid)/PEG block copolymer micelles carrying folate residues on their surface were shown to be efficient for the delivery of adriamycin to tumor cells in vitro, demonstrating the potential for solid tumor treatment and combined targetability and pH sensitivity.

The search for new ligands for cancer targeting concentrates around specific receptors overexpressed on cancer cells. Thus, liposome targeting to tumors has been achieved by using vitamin and growth factor receptors. Vasoactive intestinal peptide (VIP) was used to target PEG liposomes with radionuclides to VIP receptors of the tumor, which enhanced breast cancer inhibition in rats. PEG liposomes were targeted by arginine-glycine-aspartate peptides to integrins of tumor vasculature and, being loaded with doxorubicin, demonstrated increased efficiency against C26 colon carcinoma in a murine model. A similar angiogenic homing peptide was used for targeted delivery to vascular endothelium of drug-loaded liposomes in experimental treatment of tumors in mice.

Epidermal growth factor receptor (EGFR)-targeted immunoliposomes were delivered to a variety of tumor cells overexpressing EGFR. Mitomycin C in long-circulating hyaluronan-targeted liposomes increases Mitomycin C activity against tumors overexpress hyaluronan receptors. Studies also continue with galactosylated liposomes used to target drugs to the liver for therapy of liver tumors or metastases. Cisplatin-loaded liposomes specifically binding chondroitin sulfate, which is overexpressed in many tumor cells, were used for successful suppression of tumor growth and metastases in vivo. Mannosylated liposomes with muramyl dipeptide significantly inhibited liver metastases in tumor-bearing mice.

8

Drug Rehabilitation and Therapy Analysis

While in treatment, individuals learn about addiction, recovery, and the dangers of relapse while simultaneously confronting misunderstandings about self, others, and their environment. A drug rehabilitation centre like Michael's House helps individual's make important lifestyle changes, manage feelings, develop tools for coping, and learn skills instrumental in successful abstinence.

Our drug rehab centres also teach individuals to identify the warning signs for drug and alcohol relapse and design effective strategies for preventing a relapse. Statistics show that without a solid plan to avoid or handle addiction triggers, patients often relapse into the behaviour that brought them to the drug rehab facility.

For many drug addicts and alcoholics, success is a direct function of the amount of assistance they receive during their rehabilitation programme. Those who remain in a drug rehab centre longer than three months usually have better results than those who spend less time there. Research conducted over the last 25 years demonstrates that drug rehabilitation centres work to reduce an individual's drug use as well as prevent the potential commission of crimes by drug abusers. Research has also shown that those who have successfully completed a drug rehab programme are more likely to secure employment.

For most individuals, an inpatient residential drug rehab programme is the best option for successful recovery. Research indicates that inpatient drug rehab is the most successful kind of care for those who have had multiple unsuccessful attempts at recovery through outpatient treatment. Those who have abused drugs or alcohol heavily for years may have even more difficulty quitting.

An individual in this category may be best served by attending a long-term inpatient alcohol and drug rehab programme like our Extended Care Program. A drug rehab centre's ability to handle all types of drug addiction is critical. At Michael's House we understand how to detox and treat specific drug addictions such as: methamphetamine addiction, marijuana addiction, heroin addiction, cocaine addiction, xanax abuse, and prescription medication abuse.

NATIONAL SCENARIO OF DRUG ADDICTION

Pakistan has long been exposed to the consequences of illicit opium cultivation,, production, trafficking and abuse. The extent and gravity of the problem has, however, fluctuated over time. The use of certain opium poppy and cannabis products has a long history and has acquired a degree of psychological and socio-cultural acceptance.

Falling in a region that produces nearly 90 percent of the world's opiates, Pakistan is facing multi dimensional threats emerging from its being the most favorite drug route, re-cultivation of poppy, smuggling of precursors and psychotropic substances and an alarming increase in its population of drug addicts. Now the drug menace is spreading into previously an affected area, fresh gangs are emerging, and new trafficking rates and drugs of abuse, particularly synthetics and solvents, are being discovered.

The drug abuse scenario in Pakistan is likely to worsen if assessed against the backdrop of the steep rise in poppy cultivation and production of heroin in Afghanistan. A major chunk of the heroin produced in Afghanistan is finding its way into Iran and Pakistan-both for local consumption as well as for illegal export through land and sea routes. However, Pakistan is faced with a serious dilemma.

In view of its international commitments, it must implement stringent anti-smuggling measures at its borders; this measure has the potential to be accompanied by the looming danger of increased availability of heroin on the streets. It is, therefore, necessary to halt cultivation and production of heroin in the source country so that the drug does not find its way into neighboring countries, like Pakistan, Iran and Central Asian Republics, where existing resources constraints make it impossible for these countries to allocate additional resources to deal with the situation. At the same time, increase in local consumption would lead to a cyclic increase in production and narcotics money, which can be reinvested to fund heroin exports to relatively more lucrative markets in the west.

Cultivation

Pakistan is facing a serious and complex situation in narcotics. Two narcotics plants (i) the opium poppy and (ii) cannabis have traditionally been growth in Pakistan. Cannabis grows wild in most parts in Pakistan and as a cultivated plant in the north of the country.

The irresistible temptation to collect and convert it into cannabis resin (charas and hashish) for sale and easy profit is thus understandable. In recent times, poppy cultivation was restricted to three types of administratively diverse areas in the, Khyber Pakhtoon Khawa(KPK) strategically very important and politically very sensitive because of their close proximity to the Afghan and Soviet borders. These are (a) settled districts, (b) merged areas or Provincially Administered Tribal Areas (PATA) and (c) Federally Administered Tribal Areas (FATA).

The cultivation of poppy in the merged or PATA which at one time accounted for about 20% of opium production in Pakistan, now accounts for all of the opium produced in Pakistan. These areas were not governed by a licensing system or any central law enforcement agency; and presently the national laws of the country are being gradually extended to them in a phased manner. The FATA, which contributed today 40-50% of the total production of opium, enjoy a special status, as they continue to be largely administered by tribal custom and tradition.

In 2003 poppy cultivation was reported at 6,703 ha. Which included opium production in Balochistan, the Khyber Pakhtoon Khawa (KPK) and the Federally Administered Tribal Areas (FATA). Poppy cultivation in Balochistan was reported for the first time in 2003; most of the poppy cultivated in Balochistan has been eradicated every year since then. Over the past three years the Khyber Agency (on the border with Nangarhar province in Afghanistan) in the FATA has harvested the bulk of opium around 1.2 percent of the area cultivated in Afghanistan, there is a risk that cultivation in Pakistan could increase substantially unless there are sustained efforts to dissuade farmers from planting poppy and to destroy opium crops before they are harvested (UNODC, 2010).

Due to sincere efforts of the government the country was able to achieve poppy-free status in 2000. In spite of the re-emergence of poppy cultivation in the last two yeas Pakistan is not producing heroine due to timely destruction of poppy crops by law enforcement agencies and strict surveillance to prevent the establishment of heroine laboratories on the country's soil, but poppy cultivation has resumed in the country, though on a small scale according to the new report of International Narcotic Control Board in 2006, "poppy's now cultivated in parts of southern province of Balochistan, Districts of Khyber Agency and Kohistan in KPK.

Lack of monitoring and eradication combined with poverty remain the key reasons for the re-emergence of opium cultivation. Efforts to stem opium cultivation in neighboring Afghanistan and also forced some growers across the border" (UNODCP, 2002).

Trafficking

Narcotics production and refining in Afghanistan is a major impact on Pakistan. According to the UNODC's Afghanistan Opium Survey 2007, around 70% of Afghanistan's opium was grown in five provinces along the border with Pakistan includes Kandahar, Nirmoz, Nangarhar, Badakhshan and Helmand. Pakistan geographical condition provides a favorable corridor for trafficking (UNODCP, 2002).

The ANF (Anti-Narcotics Force) has identified the following trends in the trafficking of illicit drugs through Pakistan Trafficking through unaccompanied baggage; Impregnated letters/soaked apparels; Trafficking of liquid heroin; Hiring of families as couriers; Use of air courier services Convoys through Balochistan, Increased resistance to interdiction efforts; Night movement use of Satellite phones for coordination Through airports trend are concealment in baggage, Concealment by swallowing/ingesting concealment by wrapping around bodies Heroin concealed in shampoo bottles; Increased trafficking of psychotropic injections. The common trends through seaports are trafficking using container Increased trafficking using boats.

The porous borders in between Pakistan and Afghanistan facilitate trafficking of afghan drugs to various parts of the world through Pakistan. This situation enhances the vulnerability as a transit corridor. Open and scarcely inhabited areas of Baluchistan especially near Zhob, Chaman, Taftan, Mand and Makran coast facilitate trafficking of drugs through vehicular convoys and animal transport from southern Afghanistan. These areas also provide dumping sites foe the drugs before these are trafficked beyond Pakistan.

After crossing the Afghanistan Pakistan (Baluchistan) border same drugs are transported across the Iranian province of Sistan, Balochistan for onward movement towards turkey and Western Europe. The coastal areas of Pakistan,(including Karachi, Port Qasim, and the small fishing ports along Makran costal), Are also vulnerable to drug smuggling activities towards gulf states and beyond large hasish seizires effected in the province of Khyber Pakhtoon Khuwa (KPK) indicates that hasish is also smuggled from Afghanistan through FATA and then further trafficked to coastal areas using land routes, from where it is shipped abroad. Similarly heroin seizures pattern suggests the large quantities are transit through KPK/FATA, from where it is trafficked to world destination using air and sea routes.

Consumption

Pakistan is the second largest country in the south Asia region with an estimated population of 170 million. It's demographic and health profile is similar to the rest of South Asian countries, characterized by the high rates of infant and maternal mortality, low level of literacy and poor access to health care. Additionally, already crunched health budget is being diluted due to expenditure on burgeoning problem of drug of dependence HIV/AIDS caused by use of injecting drug. Drug abuse study surveys conducted in 1980, 1982,1988,1993,2000 and 2006 indicate the increase in number of drug abuse at the rate of 7% annually.

The 2006 National Assessment Report on Problem Drug Use in Pakistan estimates that there are 628,000 opiate users. Of these, around 482,000 (77 percent) are heroin users. Given the massive increase of opium and heroin production in Afghanistan, the relative stability in the numbers of the opiate abusing population over the past six yeas is a notable achievement.

However, the number of injecting drug users (IDUs) in 2006 is estimated at 125,000, double the estimated figure for 2000. This is a cause for concern particularly in terms of the HIV/AIDS transmission risk (UNODC. 2006).

The prevalence rates for opiate use range from 0.4 percent in the provinces of Punjab and Sindh to 0.7 percent in the KPK and 1.1 percent in Balochistan. The latter two provinces share a direct border with Afghanistan. While the overall rate of abuse has not changed much in Pakistan, the proportion of drug users who inject has increased from 15 percent in 2000 to 29 percent in 2006 (UNODC. 2006).

According to the 2006 National Assessment Report, the majority of opiate users (77%) were using heroin while the remainder were using opium and other opiates. Most of the opiate users were multiple users, i.e., they were using more than one substance at any given time or during a day. Many drug users reported facing serious health and social problems. Around 8 percent reported having HIV infection, 18 percent reported having Tuberculosis and 11 percent reported Hepatitis C infection.

The report estimates the average age of opiate users at 35.5 years. Countrywide, up to 33 percent of the drug users were between 31 to 40 years old, while in Punjab and Singh up to 40 percent of the drug users were between 16 and 30 years old. The majority of opiate users (72 percent) were still living at home. While 38 percent had no education, 25 percent had up to primary and one third up to high school education. Around one third of the opiate users were unemployed, while the remainder had been supporting them through casual work (39 percent), or had been working part or full time (15 percent and 7 percent respectively). Therefore, contrary to conventional assumptions, a significant proportion of opiate users can and do participate in economic activity (UNODC. 2006).

Situation in Neighboring Countries

The successful ban imposed on opium poppy cultivation in Afghanistan on July 2000, was recognized at the international level but the reprieve was short lived as cultivation resumed on a large scale in 2002, spiraling from 185 metric tons to 3,400 metric tons and registering a further increase by 8% in 2003 i.e. 3,600 metric tons. In 2004, opium poppy cultivation increased by 2/ 3, reaching an unprecedented 131,000 hectors, as reported in the 2004 Afghanistan opium survey of the United Nations Office on Drugs and Crimes (UNODC). Cultivation stretched across all 32 provinces, making the illicit industry the engine of economic growth and the strongest link of the Afghan nation. At present, the opium economy is valued US$ 2.8 billions, equivalent to about 60% of Afghan GDP. The opium economy involves 2.3 million people meaning one in 10 of the Afghan population (UNODC. 2010).

It caters to 90% of the world's demand for opium and heroin. Being in close proximity of Afghanistan, all regional countries, especially Pakistan, are being extensively used for the transit of Afghan opiates. It's estimated that opium production in 2007, 2008, and 2009 stud at 8200, 7700 and 6900 metric tons respectively. Approximately 56% of total opium production estimated to be smuggled as morphine and heroin. It is also believed that 40 percent Afghan opiates are smuggled through/ into Pakistan. Cannabis is grown as cash crops especially in the northern region of Afghanistan. UNODC carried out first comprehensive survey in Afghanistan in 2009 and reported cultivation of approx. 20,000 to 25,000 hectors (UNODC. 2009).

With the increase in trafficking through Pakistan, the availability of Afghan drug also increased in the country correspondingly. The situation was aggravated by the inflow of Afghan opium in the tribal areas of Pakistan from across the border. The presence of mobile groups among the 3 million refugees further complicated the affairs.

The consumption of opium and heroin has increased along the drug trafficking routes, which are constantly proliferating. Numerous new routes have emerged other than the historical Balkan route connecting Afghanistan, Pakistan, Iran, Turkey and Europe.

The Iran is situated in Middle East, bordering the Gulf of Oman, the Persian Gulf and Caspian Sea between Iran and Pakistan. The population of Iran is 65,875,224 (2008) and the adult prevalence rate of HIV/AIDS is 0.2% in 2005. On the other hand people living with HIV/AIDS, 66,000 in 2005 (UNODC. 2009).

Despite substantial interdiction efforts and considerable control measures along the border with Afghanistan, Iran remains one of the primary transshipment routes for Southwest Asian heroin to Europe; suffers one of the highest opiate addiction rates in the world, and has an increasing problem with synthetic drugs; lacks anti-money laundering laws; has reached out to neighboring countries to share counter-drug intelligence

The region constituting Pakistan, Afghanistan, Iran and the Central Asian Republic has been witnessing the rise and fall of poppy cultivation for the last many decades. This fluctuation has had ramifications on the socio-political milieu of these countries. Pakistan earned the status of a "poppy-free country" in 2001-02 but the 2002-03 and 2003-04 crops seasons were again marked by resumption of opium much to the detriment of the country's had earned status (UNODC. 2009).

The drug abuse scenario in Pakistan is likely to worsen if assessed against the backdrop of the steep rise in poppy cultivation and production of heroin in Afghanistan. A major chunk of the heroin produced in Afghanistan is finding its way into Iran and Pakistan-both for local consumption as well as for illegal export through land and sea routes.

The region constituting Pakistan, Afghanistan, Iran and the Central Asian Republic has been witnessing the rise and fall of poppy cultivation for the last many decades. This fluctuation has had ramifications on the socio-political milieu of these countries. Pakistan earned the status of a "poppy-free country" in 2001-02 but the 2002-03 and 2003-04 crops seasons were again marked by resumption of opium much to the detriment of the country's had earned status.

THERAPY ANALYSIS - DRUG ADDICTION

Rewarding Behaviour, But at What Cost?

The neurochemistry associated with drug use and addiction is complex and involves many interrelated pathways. However, all drugs of addiction have one thing in common - they produce a sensation in the user that is pleasurable, the so-called 'high'. The common factor for all abused drugs is that they stimulate the mesolimbic reward pathway in the brain, with the neurotransmitter dopamine a key element. This chemical is released naturally by the brain in response to stimuli such as food or sex, but it is also released by drugs of abuse. Substances which activate the reward pathway are positively reinforcing - that is to say, the pleasurable effects experienced by the user when the pathway is stimulated drives them to repeat the experience. It is when this reinforcement becomes aberrant and the user engages in compulsive drugseeking behaviour, that true addiction sets in. To compound the problem, tolerance to the effects of a drug builds up over time, often by the reduction in dopamine receptors on the dendrites of neurons. The user therefore requires more and more to achieve the desired effects and when the drug is no longer available, such as when an effort is made to quit, an addict will go through a period of withdrawal. The overstimulated reward pathway is no longer active and a dysphoric state ensues. This often leads to relapse.

...Perhaps the most addictive of drugs is cocaine, which is linked to not only the dopamine pathway of the midbrain, but also the glutamate and the noradrenaline pathway...

The involvement of neurotransmitters has been explored scientifically throughout the last century and many scientists now implicate the neurotransmitters 5- HT (serotonin), noradrenaline and glutamate in the process of addiction. Perhaps the most addictive of drugs is cocaine, which is linked to not only the dopamine pathway of the midbrain, but also the glutamate and the noradrenaline pathway, which activates the fight-or-flight response triggering an increase in heart rate, blood pressure, body temperature and dilation of the pupils. Cocaine binds to the dopamine reuptake transporters, thus blocking functionality and as a result, dopamine levels increase in the synapse, so the receiving neuron is continuously stimulated - this constant firing of the neurons leads to a feeling of euphoria. Another factor in the reinforcement of cocaine use lies in the fact that after cocaine administration, dopamine levels fall significantly below normal, pre-consumption levels. The user therefore feels a "low", and the immediate response to alleviate this low is to consume more cocaine to raise the level once again. Being a key player in memory regulation, it is theorized that glutamate is directly linked to trigger memories that lead to relapse. In one study, researchers stimulated a memory-related brain area that is rich with glutamate, which caused rats weaned off of cocaine to frantically press a lever that previously dispensed the drug. In essence it caused a relapse, and blocking glutamate activity subsequently blocked the response.

Generally, the neurochemistry of addiction is heavily theorized and not yet fully understood, and the addictive nature of drugs varies from substance to substance, and from individual to individual. Owing to their neurochemical effects, drugs such as codeine or alcohol, typically require many more exposures to addict their users than drugs such as heroin or cocaine. Likewise, a person who is psychologically or genetically predisposed to addiction is much more likely to suffer from it. There are anecdotal reports of psychological addiction to recreational stimulants such as MDMA (ecstasy) and a dissociative psychedelic ketamine, but it is thought that pills sold on the street as 'ecstasy' often contain adulterants, which may be the addictive compound.

ROAD TO RECOVERY–DRUGS FOR DRUGS

Treatment of drug addiction is usually multifactorial, with a combination of counselling, psychotherapy and pharmacotherapy often employed, depending on the substance involved. Pharmacotherapy for drug addiction, particularly as the neurochemical basis of addiction and reward becomes further elucidated, is becoming more and more common, and below we will look at some of the various therapies available and in development for some common drug addictions. The traditional approach is to give a compound that mimics a drug's action but does not provide the same intense 'high', thus satisfying cravings and avoiding withdrawal whilst drug use can be tapered off. More novel strategies are also under investigation such as compounds and vaccines that block the activity of a drug completely. As would be expected, the pharmaceutical industry has focused most of its efforts where the biggest potential rewards are to be made.

Indeed, our data shows that of all the drugs in active development for a variety of drug addictions, it is clear that smoking is the main focus of much of this research, followed by drugs to treat alcohol addiction.

SMOKING AND ALCOHOL

Even tobacco companies no longer dispute the addictive nature of nicotine, found in all tobacco products. It leads to rapid activation of the dopamine reward system, particularly because smoking provides the perfect drug delivery vehicle. The field of smoking cessation therapies is already crowded, with multiple OTC products such as nicotine gums and patches available for the individual trying to quit. These therapies simply replace the nicotine a smoker would have received from cigarettes.

For those who fail to kick the habit using this approach, the standard non-nicotine drug therapy until recently had been a sustained-release formulation of the antidepressant buproprion, marketed as Zyban by GlaxoSmithKline. Whilst the exact mechanism by which it produces anti-smoking effects is unknown, it is a weak inhibitor of both dopamine and noradrenaline reuptake. Recently, a second drug has become available, with Pfizer's launch of Champix/ Chantix (varenicline tartrate), a partial agonist at the a4a2 nicotine receptor. Useful as these compounds are, they still only produce quit rates of less than 50%, and so drug development in this area continues apace. In late-stage trials currently are GlaxoSmithKline's GW-468816, an NMDA glycine site antagonist, and dianicline (SSR-591813), a nicotinic a4a2 partial agonist under development by Sanofi- Aventis. Using a very different approach, Celtic Pharma is developing an immunotherapy, TA-NIC. This vaccine induces production of antibodies against nicotine, thus preventing the nicotine from crossing the blood-brain barrier and hence removing the positively reinforcing effect. Acting in a similar fashion is Cytos Biotechnology's CYT002-NicQb, a nicotine vaccine in Phase II and recently partnered with Novartis.

In cases of chronic alcohol abuse, the standard drug therapy is the opioid receptor antagonist naltrexone (which is also used to treat opiate addiction). It has been shown to reduce the frequency and severity of relapse to drinking, mediated, it is presumed, through modulation of the dopaminergic system usually activated by ethanol. A sustained-release formulation of naltrexone developed by Alkermes is also just becoming available in various markets, and BioTie's nalmefene tablet formulation is also waiting in the wings. A second drug currently prescribed for alcohol addiction is acamprosate. This acts in a very different way - it increases GABA-ergic transmission in the brain through the inhibition of EAA receptors. Much further back in the pipeline, CV Therapeutics is developing an aldehyde dehydrogenase 2 antagonist for the treatment of alcohol dependence, which is hoped to be an improvement on standard aversion therapy drugs such as disulfiram.

NARCOTICS

The opiate narcotic heroin (the street name of diamorphine) activates mu opioid receptors in the brain that are usually activated by endogenous substances. The stimulation of these opioid receptors from heroin leads to feelings of intense euphoria, known as a rush, accompanied with flushing of the skin, and heavy extremities. This is also linked to an increase in the neuronal firing of dopaminergic cells. Following this rush, the user experiences an alternately wakeful and drowsy state due to the clouding of mental functioning due to the depression of the central nervous system.

Long-term effects occur after a long period of repeated use, and chronic users may develop infection of the heart lining and valves, abscesses, collapsed veins and liver disease. In a similar way to other drugs, mainly cocaine, repeated heroin use is triggered by its often devastating physical withdrawal effects. This withdrawal may occur as early as a few hours after the last administration in regular abusers and includes restlessness, muscle and bone pain, insomnia, cold flashes with goose bumps, kicking movements and diarrhoea and vomiting, which all produce drug craving.

In addition to the use of a replacement therapy, such as methadone, opioid antagonists such as naltrexone are commonly used to treat opiate addiction. Currently in Phase III trials for the 6mth treatment of opioid addiction is Titan Pharmaceuticals' subcutaneous formulation of buprenorphine, Probuphine, and Indevus has an extended release formulation of naltrexone in Phase II trials.

COCAINE AND METHAMFETAMINE

As explained previously, cocaine inhibits the reuptake of dopamine, increasing the availability of dopamine in the synapse and increasing dopamine's action on the postsynaptic neurons. The 'high' is short-lived, meaning that users repeatedly administer cocaine to repeat the effect. Methamfetamine is a dopaminergic and adrenergic reuptake inhibitor. It rapidly enters the brain causing a cascading release of norepinephrine, dopamine and 5-HT. Both cocaine and methamfetamine use is on the rise in the Western world, which would suggest that these drug addictions may soon be more on the radar of the pharmaceutical industry. At present, there are no drugs specifically approved for the treatment of these addictions, and the usual approach is to administer drugs to deal with the effects of the different phases of withdrawal, such as sedatives or antidepressants, and offer counselling. Similar to its nicotine vaccine discussed above, Celtic Pharma is also developing a vaccine against cocaine use, TA-CD that has reached Phase II development. For methamfetamine addiction, Yaupon Therapeutics is collaborating with the US NIH on the development of the first specific pharmacological treatment - an alkaloid from Indian tobacco called lobeline.

THE FUTURE?

The development pipeline for pharmacotherapeutics for drug addiction (Graph 1) shows that there are many companies active in this area, including some traditional big pharma such as Pfizer, Eli Lilly and Merck KGaA, as well as a host of small-to-middle size pharma and biotech enterprises. Indeed, no one company dominates the area and there is still much room for improvement over existing therapies. As has been seen, much of the research is currently focused on improved formulations of existing drugs. With drug use a continuing social and economic problem worldwide, it is hoped that as the mechanisms of addiction are further elucidated, new pharmacological strategies will be developed

LOVE FIRST: INTERVENTION FOR ALCOHOLISM AND DRUG ADDICTION

One out of three people is living with or related to someone with an alcohol or other drug problem, and intervention can get these people into treatment. Alcoholics and addicts are also our family members and friends. Although we see their problem, they cannot. When we offer help, they refuse. When we talk to them, they blame us or someone else. It begins to feel hopeless, but it is not. This website will show you how to take action. Intervention teaches families and friends a language alcoholics can understand. It organizes love and honesty in a way that breaks through denial. It creates a moment of clarity for the alcoholic. Most people suffering from alcoholism and drug addiction will accept help on intervention day. You can meet our professional interventionists here.

Intervention requires new information. Learn for yourself, then ask other family members to join you. Once everyone is educated, you can make a family decision about intervention. If you decide to move ahead, planning and preparation are your keys to success. Take no shortcuts. We are able to address problems with alcoholism, drug addiction, dual diagnosis, sex addiction, eating disorders, gambling addiction and other compulsive disorders.

Jeff Jay and Debra Jay are professional interventionists and authors. They will answer your brief questions about alcoholism and chemical dependency personally via e-mail. You may also arrange for a professional consultation by telephone. Debra Jay has been seen frequently on the Oprah Winfrey Show, and Jeff Jay has been seen recently on the Jane Pauley Show. Alcohol and other drug intervention opens the door to treatment and recovery. People rebuild their lives. Families rebuild relationships. Children heal and learn to trust again. Change begins by simply doing the next right thing.

Information on the Web site is based on the Hazelden Guidebook, Love First: A New Approach to Intervention for Alcoholism and Drug Addiction, by Jeff Jay and Debra Jay (Hazelden, 2000). Click on the title to read what people are saying about Love First. Former senator George McGovern, who lost his daughter Terry to alcoholism, writes the foreword.

Family Intervention

Family intervention is a method that uses the power of love and concern to break through denial and get a person into treatment. By organizing family members and friends in a very specific way, we are able to get results that were impossible in the past. Here's an excerpt from the best-selling book on intervention, Love First, by Jeff Jay and Debra Jay:

"Intervention is the most effective technique families can use to help a loved one suffering from chemical dependency —alcoholism or other drug addiction. It is also the most ignored. But just as CPR is often the first, life saving step in helping a heart attack victim, intervention is the most powerful step that a family can take to initiate the recovery process. "There are many common misconceptions about intervention. Some think it is an emotional ambush or an uncaring attack. But Love First demonstrates that intervention is a carefully planned process founded on love and honesty. Many people have heard about tough love where tough comes first; this book puts love first.

"Through our work in intervention, we have found that love is a powerful force when confronting addiction. In the past, expressions of love were delegated to a few brief sentences during an intervention. We've learned that when we expand the role of love in intervention, it is love that first breaks through denial, not toughness. Using love first, we often never have to use tough love."

The keys to a successful intervention are planning, preparation and technique. Many families think they've tried everything, but on closer examination their best efforts have failed because they've been unwittingly working against each other. The alcoholic or addict often plays one person off against another, keeping the family off balance.

Intervention unifies the family and gets everyone working together. Before the intervention ever takes place, the team goes through a planning a rehearsal process that leaves nothing to chance. For example, here is an intervention checklist. A family intervention begins with one person looking for a way to end the problems caused by alcoholism or other addictions.

Those who love the alcoholic put aside everything they think they know, and begin anew. With a thorough and updated education, the family makes a well-informed decision about intervention. There are several ways to educate yourself on intervention. You can hire a professional interventionist to guide the family. The interventionist will help you decide if intervention is right for your family and how best to help affected children. He or she will also lead the intervention.

To find an interventionist in your hometown, call a local alcohol and drug treatment centre. If none is available locally, call a nationally recognized treatment centre like Hazelden that maintains a list of interventionists who work nationwide. When contacting an interventionist outside your hometown, ask if he or she offers initial family consultations via telephone conferencing calls. You may also contact us to inquire about our pessional intervention services.

You can also educate yourselves using low-cost resources on intervention. You can get the best-selling book Love First from almost any library or bookstore — it is very wideley available. If you need a professional later, you can make the investment then. We also offer a comprehensive online video course on intervention. This method will take you step-by-step through the whole process, using streaming video. You can watch the video right now on your computer for about the cost of one hour of clinical treatment. To learn more, click here. Once family members and close friends understand that intervention is based on love and dignity, it is likely they will support taking this well-planned, highly successful approach to helping a loved one. How do you know? If you're not sure if your loved one has a problem with alcohol or other drugs, take this quiz.

Choose How You Want to Take Action

Knowledge is power when dealing with addiction. Planning and preparation are critical for a good, structured family intervention. These four options range from simple reading to hiring a professional interventionist. Choose the method that's right for you.

1. *Start Learning:* This website is loaded with information about addiction, recovery, intervention, treatment and more. You might want to start by reading the page on

   You can learn a great deal about how to help your loved one, just by reading through our website.

2. *Get the Directions: Love First* is the best-selling book on intervention. It will take you step-by-step through the process of planning and carrying out a good structured family intervention. It will help you get your loved on into treatment.

   The authors, Jeff Jay and Debra Jay, explain the dynamics of addiction, the process of enabling, choosing a team, writing intervention letters, and all the steps families need to know to carry out a good, structured intervention. Love First is available in almost any bookstore, or you can buy it on amazon.com by clicking here.

"Building a team, choosing a chairperson, anticipating objections, using checklists, and rehearsing for the intervention itself. The reader will find it all here!" -Robert M. Morse, M.D., Professor of psychiatry emeritus, Mayo Medical School former Director of Addictive Disorders Services, Mayo Clinic

3. *Watch the Intervention Workshop Videos:* Jeff and Debra Jay have produced a comprehensive video series that will teach you how to plan and carry out a powerful family intervention. These videos are available to watch immediately over the internet (like YouTube). For more information and to watch sample videos, click here.

   This moderately priced option is almost like having Jeff and Debra Jay work with you personally. The Workshop is presented in 38 separate video chapters for easy viewing. To learn more about Intervention Workshop, just click here.

4. *Hire a Professional Interventionist:* Whether you want a brief consultation and strategy session by phone or a professionally facilitated intervention from start to finish, we are ready to help you.

Jeff and Debra Jay and their team of intervention specialists help families every day. Read about our professional background. We are available to discuss your case and/or travel to your location now. Most families take a week or two to plan and carry out an intervention with us. But we can also intervene in as little as 24 hours, if necessary.

A group of Chinese scientists has discovered the main biochemical pathways in drug addiction—and without having to do a single experiment. Modern biology has a lot of "omes". The genome—all the genes that go to make up an organism—is a familiar idea. The proteome—all the different proteins—is becoming so. But there are also the transcriptome (RNA), the glycome (sugars), the lipidome (fats) and the metabolome (all the miscellaneous odds and ends not covered by the others). And then there is the bibliome—all the mentions in research papers of known biomolecules. There are now so many of these papers, and the databases linking them are so good, that it is possible to use scientific methods to investigate the bibliome in its own right, just as any of the other, wetter "omes" may be investigated. Which is exactly what a group of researchers from Peking University, led by Wei Liping, have done to get at the biochemical heart of drug addiction.

Dr Wei and her colleagues wanted to answer three questions. First, what are the genes and biochemical pathways in addiction? Second, does addiction to different substances involve the same core biochemical mechanisms? Third, does anything in those mechanisms explain why addiction is so hard to shake off? Many people, of course, have asked these questions before, and partial answers have emerged. What Dr Wei hoped to do was to take these fragmentary answers and patch them together to make something approaching the whole truth. And, in a paper just published in the *Public Library of Science*, she seems to have managed just that.

It Looks Good on Paper

Dr Wei's group looked at more than 1,000 studies of the biochemistry and genetics of drug addiction. They were interested in the four sorts of drug reckoned most addictive: alcohol, cocaine, nicotine and opiates (heroin, methadone and so on).

About 1,500 genes were implicated by one or more of the studies, but in only 396 cases was that implication backed by at least two independent lines of evidence. It was on these confirmed cases that Dr Wei concentrated her fire.

Biochemistry is about pathways and networks of pathways. A pathway is a series of enzymes (each of which is encoded in a gene) that perform a task in sequence, like workers on an assembly line. Dr Wei therefore ran her 396 genes through a database of all known pathways to see which involved several enzymes encoded by those genes. She found 18 that were involved in addiction to at least one type of drug. Five, however, were common to all four types, and these five pathways therefore look as though they are at the core of the process of addiction. Three of the five were already under suspicion. Dr Wei's result provided strong statistical evidence to back up what had just been hunches. Two other pathways, however, had not previously been considered as being involved in addiction.

The existence of these five central pathways helps explain a lot about addiction.

First, it gives weight to the belief that some people are more susceptible to all sorts of addiction than others are. That contrasts with the thought that addictions are substance-by-substance phenomena, though the two ideas are not mutually exclusive since changes in the 13 substance-specific pathways clearly also result in addiction.

Second, the particular pathways involved help to explain why addiction is so hard to reverse. Several of them take part in strengthening the connections between nerve cells, which is the underlying basis of learning. Unlearning something by breaking these connections is hard.

Third, Dr Wei was able to link the five central pathways together into a network, and show that this network has four positive-feedback loops in it. Work on other species in other contexts suggests that the mixture of loops she found was one that often results in rapid and irreversible biological processes—which is exactly what is seen in addiction.

None of this, of course, directly helps the addict, though it reinforces the message that it is better not to start taking these drugs in the first place. But working out how the addiction machine operates may point those looking for therapies in the right direction. And this study also shows that the old cry "more research is necessary" is not always true. Sometimes all you need to do is look at what you already have in a different way.

OPIATE ADDICTION VS. OPIATE DEPENDENCY

You did not choose to become addicted. Opiate dependency, like any prescription medication dependency, has turned many back surgery and chronic pain patients into what the medical community calls 'accidental addicts'.

The Waismann Method^{sm} of Rapid Detoxification offers a humane treatment to individuals physically dependent on opiate drugs. Many patients who come to us started out treating their neck pain, back pain, migraine headaches, or other musculoskeletal disorders at normal doses. Gradually, self-medication progressed to excessive levels as a means also to avoid withdrawal. Our experts in pain management evaluate post-procedure care for persons dependent on opiate prescription painkillers such as OxyContin ®, Vicodin ®, Darvocet ®, and Percocet ®, among others.

Persons with opiate dependency may experience the same symptoms and withdrawal—but not necessarily the same social behaviour—as so-called 'drug addicts'. "After a crushed spine, many surgeries, and 12 years using doctor-prescribed drugs," says opiate detox patient Scott, "it was very hard to break free." "My life was horrible. I was not in control because of opiates. The drugs ran my entire life. I could not plan anything, nor go anywhere without knowing where the drugs were and if I had enough. I became scared of the withdrawals, worse than anything." Opiate dependency afflicts people from all walks of life, regardless of social or economic status—homemakers, stockbrokers, athletes, entertainers, skilled laborers, students, and others like yourself.

Opiate Addiction Treatment and Opiate Dependency Treatment

Thanks to the Waismann Method ^{sm} of Rapid Detox programme, states Scott, "...You gave me a fighting chance to make it, in the most humane way as possible with modern medicine."

Anesthesia Assisted Medical Opiate Detoxification (Rapid Detox) frees you from the cycle of dependency. The Waismann Method of Rapid Detox is a world-renowned treatment for flushing opiate toxins out of a drug dependent body. Board Certified doctors treat and monitor suffering in-patients:

- Patients sleep comfortably throughout the procedure, unaware of discomfort from opiate withdrawal.
- ICU staff monitor patients through their recovery during the procedure.
- Patients leave the hospital opiate-free, without other opiate-based replacement drugs like Subutex, Suboxone, or Methadone.
- Post-treatment patients can reclaim their lives within a short period of time.

The Waismann Method sm of Rapid Detox from Opiate Dependency. What you should know about Rapid Detox and The Waismann Method:

- Ours is the most reputed and thorough detox treatment in the country .
- Our doctors have unsurpassed experience in treating opiate patients under anesthesia (Rapid Detox).
- We originated and first brought The Waismann Method to North America ten years ago.
- Our patients undergo thorough, individual medical pre-screening.
- We have treated the highest levels of opiate intake in the country—substitutions or lower dosage not required before procedure.
- Our supervising physicians are programme-dedicated specialists (not residency staff).
- The Waismann Method provides the highest success rate in the field of opiate dependency.
- Procedure requires minimal anesthesia (1-11/2 hours) for maximal safety protocol
- Patients receive the utmost level of care in an accredited hospital setting (not out-patient clinic) over 4-5 days.
- Protocol assures unparalleled safety via cardiology and radiology assessments, diagnostic tests, Board Certified Anesthesiologists, pain and other indicated specialists.
- Unique and completely opiate-free treatment offers safe and most humane method.
- Within a decade, thousands of patients from all over the world have detoxified.

- More and more patients come to us lately from other rehab or drug detox centres, which promised them detoxification but instead provided them addictive replacement drugs like Suboxone!
- Follow-up services offer individually-tailored retreat and after-care programmes.

Opiate dependency was not your choice when you originally sought pain relief. But opiate addiction detoxification and new freedom can be yours. Some rapid detox centres prescribe Suboxone, an opiate itself, as an opiate replacement, which can be as highly addictive with extended use.. The Waismann Method relies on board certified anesthesiologists within the ICU of full service hospital, so that if any medical assistance is required it is immediately on hand.

MICHAEL'S HOUSE

Measuring Success One Miracle At a Time

Michael's House is nationally recognized for providing effective drug rehab and alcohol rehab treatment for individuals and families suffering from the disease of alcoholism, substance abuse as well as co-occurring disorders.

Our two rehab centres, The Treatment Centre for Men and the Residential Retreat, are nestled in the Foothills of the magnificent San Jacinto Mountains in Palm Springs, California. Our residential rehabilitation centre and extended care facilities offer Drug Rehab, alcohol rehab, and Co-Occurring Disorder Treatment in tranquil hacienda style desert retreats that reflect our holistic philosophy of care.

Michael's House provides a simple, brief admission process to determine the length and type of addiction treatment and mental health treatment appropriate for each person's needs. We consider each individual's current situation and their history, including: types of illnesses, overall condition, life skills needed and personal goals, to ensure an optimal recovery.

When you, a loved one, or a client is sick and dealing with the diseases of addiction and/or mental illness, getting help is critical. The decision about whether to seek alcohol rehab or drug rehab is very important and is an essential part of beginning recovery. Do you or a loved one need help? Our Call Centre is available 24 hours a day to answer your questions and help with the admissions process. You may also send a confidential e-mail or have a secure, private Live Chat with a representative. We understand alcohol and drug addiction, drug rehab, and emotional and psychological conditions that can lead to despair, anxiety, depression, and thoughts of suicide. We are here to help you. We are experts who care.

THE IMPACT OF DRUG ABUSE

Family and Community

Fast-paced social, economic and technological changes present a challenge to the stability and influence of the family. The family is often viewed as the basic source of strength, providing nurturance and support for its individual members as well as ensuring stability and generational continuity for the community and culture. In reality, the family is far more complex.

At least four conceptual views of the family have been identified:

(1) First, it may be seen as protecting and sustaining both strong and weak members, helping them to deal with stress and pathology while nurturing younger and more vulnerable members.

(2) Secondly, the family may be a source of tension, problems and pathology, influencing weaker members in harmful ways, including destructive drug or alcohol use.

(3) Thirdly, it may be viewed as a mechanism for family members to interact with broader social and community groups, such as peer groups, schools, work colleagues and supervisors and persons associated with religious institutions.

(4) Fourthly, the family may be seen as an important point of intervention—a natural organizational unit for transferring and building social and community values.

Rapid social, economic and technological change may, under certain circumstances, weaken the sense of family and reduce the sense of belonging to other people, groups and places. Stability of relationships, environment and expectations is a powerful force in helping people manage their lives, especially important for children and young adults. In some societies, the classical problem of balancing discipline and control of children with nurturing support to encourage their exploration, understanding of the world and self-realisation may be complicated by substance abuse problems as well as a wide range of other conditions.

Families can have a powerful influence on shaping the attitudes, values and behaviour of children, but how do they compare with peers in terms of influence on drug taking? The influence of peer groups, which is usually strong during formative years of youth, may be stronger than that of parents in some cases. One researcher has found that friends are more similar in their use of marijuana than in any other activity or attitude. In this situation, drug use by peers may exert a greater influence than the attitudes of parents. This researcher observed that peer and parental influences are synergistic, with the highest rates of marijuana use being observed among adolescents whose parents and friends were drug users. Other investigators, however, have found that peers have a high degree of influence only when the parents have abdicated their traditional supervisory roles.

Hence, parents exercising traditional family roles may be able to limit the influence of peer groups on children's attitudes towards drug use and therefore have a crucial influence on children's behaviour. Prevention of drug problems can employ knowledge about family dynamics to address personal and social concerns of family members that otherwise would lead to drug abuse, both with respect to dysfunctional as well as intact families.

In this regard, it is important to avoid assuming "... either that parents are invariably responsible for the problems experienced by their children or that substance users can be blamed for all the problems experienced by the families in which they live".

Family factors that may lead to or intensify drug use are thought to include prolonged or traumatic parental absence, harsh discipline, failure to communicate on an emotional level, chaotic or disturbed members and parental use of drugs, which provides a negative role model for children. Lack of household stability, income or employment for a parent may increase stress on the family and its vulnerability, pushing marginal individuals to find "solutions" or solace in alcohol or drugs. Single-parent families may have increased difficulties, with the single parent being forced to function beyond his or her ability. Alcohol abuse, other substance abuse and psychopathology have been studied among family members. It is well known that having biological relatives with alcoholism increases the risk in unaffected individuals.

Also, families with histories of psychological and social pathology may be at increased risk for alcohol problems. The degree to which similar processes apply to other drugs is not as well established. Persons who are heavy users of alcohol or other drugs may show psychiatric symptoms such as depression. Dysfunctional drug or alcohol use may mask an underlying emotional illness. A frequent finding from clinical assessment of users is a "dual diagnosis", where two or more clinical conditions exist at the same time in an individual. Multiple problems in the family are also very common. The existence of an addictive personality type does not appear to have been scientifically validated, but the obvious signs of troubled persons-often exhibiting multiple symptoms-are easily recognized by expert and layman alike.

Reports of disturbed family life related to drugs are frequent in the literature. In Ireland, it was found that disrupted family life appears to be a major risk factor for drug abuse among some young persons, and that as many as 10 per cent of the young people between 15 and 20 years of age in the northern part of Dublin were addicted to heroin.

In India, an increased number of heroin addicts seeking assistance at treatment centres has been reported. It has been estimated that between a half million and a million persons became addicts in the 1980s, challenging cultural traditions and services. While the family group can, under certain circumstances, be the origin of drug problems, it can also be a potent force for treatment. Family therapy has gained increased acceptance, with the defining characteristic being the simultaneous involvement of more than one member of the family in therapeutic sessions.

Many families are supported and cared for by women. They frequently have the key role in teaching the young, ensuring that health care is provided and maintaining links with and mobilizing community support when necessary. Recognition and effective utilization of women as resources for drug prevention and treatment can improve efforts to reduce both the supply and demand for drugs. Women who are not drug abusers may be affected by problems related to drug abusing men.

The problems of male partners may affect women in the form of difficulties in interpersonal relationships, instability, violence, child abuse, economic insecurity, deprivation of schooling and risk of sexually transmitted disease, including HIV infection. Limited data on the relationship between substance abuse and the health and social conditions of children are available. A report on health problems and substance use in Honduras, one of the poorest countries in the western hemisphere, with a GNP per capita of $580 in 1992.

Health

Health problems impair family life and productive employment, diminish the quality of life and may threaten survival. A comprehensive picture of worldwide health implications of drug abuse is not available. Significant country and international data, however, are available and the impact of addictive substances on health in both industrialized. The broader context of addictive substances includes tobacco, alcohol and solvents. All of these substances have several important characteristics in common.

They alter the function of the human brain and have an impact on behaviour; they are widely used throughout the world; and they burden society by increasing social and economic costs for productive enterprises and by drawing upon limited government services. The most widely used addictive substances, alcohol and tobacco, are harmful with extensive damage to the individual, family and the community. Disease, disability and dysfunction were obviously not included in the estimate in the box but would certainly increase significantly any estimate of human costs due to substance abuse. Deaths as a result of drug abuse are a major source of concern. Recent informal estimates are that perhaps 200,000 drug-injecting-related deaths may occur per annum based on the estimated size of the current world population of injecting drug abusers of approximately 5.3 million. WHO has reported as follows: "Existing data indicated a several-fold increase in drug-related deaths over the past decade.... The yearly mortality rates among intravenous drug users or drug addicts on treatment programmes ranged between one and two per cent in Europe and the United States".

WHO's examination found that, during the period of 1980 to 1988, mortality related to drugs increased in some countries and decreased in others. It decreased in Japan and Thailand and showed little change in Austria, New Zealand and former Yugoslavia. Slight increases were seen in the former Czechoslovakia, the predecessor States of Germany, the Netherlands and Spain. Steeper increases in mortality were noted in Australia, Canada, France, Italy, Poland, the United Kingdom of Great Britain and Northern Ireland and the United States.

High variability in mortality rates, however, was found within countries and from year to year. Substances commonly associated with drug abuse-related deaths are cocaine, heroin, barbiturates and amphetamines. Benzodiazepines, hallucinogens, cannabis and other substances are less frequently implicated. Combinations of drugs and alcohol were frequently noted. Although commonly used, the term "overdose" is misleading since different reactions, such as hypersensitivity, may be the real mechanism of death in some cases rather than an acute intoxication effect due to excessive amounts of the drugs.

Availability, cost, chemical contents of the drugs, preexisting and potentially life-threatening health problems and patterns of use are all factors that may play key roles in determining whether harmful effects occur in any individual case. The most widely used controlled drug, cannabis, could be associated with some fatal accidents despite its low acute toxicity. Concerning chronic use, there may be greater risks of damaging the lungs by smoking cannabis than tobacco. Commenting on the public implications of the use of addictive substances, a major health report states: "Decisions about the control of tobacco and other addictive substances are among the most important health-related choices that societies can make collectively.

In many populations, prolonged cigarette smoking is already the greatest single cause of premature death. Alcohol and other drugs also contribute to disease and disability. The damage from substance abuse is not limited to the individuals involved; others also suffer indirectly because of drunk driving, fires, passive smoking, and drug related crime and violence".

The proportion of all drug users and abusers who end up with serious health and social problems is not known. Whatever that proportion, illicit drug use more frequently results in problems or disease rather than death. Since substance abuse is not evenly spread throughout the population, it is advisable to determine the characteristics of the specific groups involved in order to plan interventions. Drug abuse may be influenced by the social-cultural milieu, the degree to which a person is part of a structured environment, his or her personal characteristics, the specific drugs involved and the circumstances of use. The earliest stages of life are a particularly vulnerable time.

Reporting on the effects of alcohol and drug abuse on foetuses in a study carried out in four Danish cities, one researcher has found that the extent of maternal drug abuse is correlated with obstetric complications and developmental characteristics of the foetus. The effects of an unstable foetal life carry over into childhood. However, with care, many of these effects can be overcome. One of the most visible impacts of harmful drug use is seen in the consequences of cocaine use on newborn infants. Experts have found that cocaine-using pregnant women have a higher rate of spontaneous abortion. Also, mothers who carried their foetus to full gestational term had infants with depressed behaviour and poor responses to stimuli. Other studies indicate that infants exposed to sedatives, stimulants or pentachlorophenol may have marked deficits. PCP and cocaine used by mothers also may interfere with the essential bonding that occurs between mother and child at birth. Other investigators have findings supporting these views.

In discussing the victims of drug abuse, a commentator notes that "maternal drug use is a substantial and apparently growing part of the problems of unhealthy newborns. The direct victim of such passive drug taking is the child, but there are indirect victims too. Drug-damaged children put burdens on already strained systems of pediatric health care and public education.

Some of the forms of damage, particularly to cognitive function and impulse control, will tend to increase crime rates when the children become adolescents and young adults. The damaged child's future schoolmates, workmates, and neighbours will all bear some of the cost". Quite apart from the direct consequences, the care of children abandoned by, or taken away from, addicted parents again implies a considerable social cost.

Probably the most widely occurring substance abuse pattern in this context is the foetal alcohol syndrome, which involves both physical and mental deficiencies that are costly to treat, often requiring both intensive initial and long-term care. The human immunodeficiency virus causes the clinical disease acquired immunodeficiency syndrome. Unknown before the 1980s, it now is an epidemic for which there is no known cure and no vaccine.

The virus is spread by sexual intercourse, contaminated blood, mother-to-child transmission during the perinatal period and use of contaminated syringes and injection equipment. The importance of each of these means of spread varies from one region of the world to another. The devastating effects of AIDS are seen most clearly in the developing world. Two-thirds of the AIDS cases, adults and children, are in Africa, where the primary means of spread is heterosexual contact. Males may acquire the virus through use of dirty injection equipment and then transmit it to female or male sex partners. Primary prevention is the only known means of slowing the spread of this virus. Early attempts to prevent transmission of the virus between addicts sharing dirty needles focused on information programmes that advised "Don't share needles or at least clean the syringe with bleach before reusing it". Recently, however, bleach baths for injection equipment have been found to be less than fully effective. Results from some of the needle exchange programmes, although less widely accepted, have been found to be positive, according to some health officials.

Peer outreach models have been used in India, the United States and elsewhere. In addition to increasing mortality, the rapid spread of AIDS, particularly in Africa, is producing a whole new class of poor, including orphans under 10 years of age who are expected to number 1 0 million or more by the turn of the century. Serious effects are expected not only in mortality but also in reduced life expectancy, sexually transmitted diseases and endemic diseases such as tuberculosis. Impaired immune systems increase vulnerability to other diseases as well. O has projected that in 2000, 2.5 million people will be newly infected with HIV, HIV prevalence will have reached 26 million, and AIDS deaths will total 1.8 million.

The impact of AIDS will depend also on fertility, mortality and other conditions. For example, in areas such as Thailand, where fertility and mortality rates are much lower than in sub-Saharan Africa, AIDS may well contribute to actual population declines over a period of 30 years or more. According to one expert, drug injecting has been identified in 80 countries and HIV infection in 52 of them.

He states: "HIV prevention must... consider interventions which help discourage drug injecting. Particularly at risk are countries in drug producing and along drug transshipment routes in South East and South West Asia, Africa, and South America. The diffusion of injecting can occur far more rapidly than the time it takes to introduce HIV prevention activities". According to this expert, drug injecting is a relatively recent phenomenon in many countries and the new diffusion of injecting is "occurring in countries which are mostly poor, and are either in drug producing areas or along drug transshipment routes. In many countries the recent rapid diffusion of injecting has been followed by major outbreaks of HIV infection, for example throughout urban, rural and hilltribe areas in Thailand, in Manipur in northcast India, Ruili in southern China, and Myanmar".

Manipur, which shares a long border with Myanmar, and Madras, India, are examples of places where rapid increases of heroin injection have taken place. Among persons who administer drugs by injection, the proportion estimated to be infected with the virus varies widely from a low range of 1-5 per cent in the United Kingdom to 20 per cent in Germany, 30 per cent in the Netherlands, 30-80 per cent in Italy, 40-60 per cent in Spain and 58 per cent in France.

As the proportion of injecting drug users who are HIV positive increases and increased numbers of them travel, the rate of spread of the virus may also increase. As one expert notes, the "most conservative predictions by public health institutions foresee increased use of illegal drugs via injection in many countries and increased transmission of HIV among people who take drugs in this way".

The relationship between the injection of drugs and HIV transmission has become a major concern in many parts of the world. But, according to a WHO report, less well "recognized, but statistically and medically more significant in terms of its overall societal impact, is the relationship between substance abuse and hepatitis, tuberculosis, cardiovascular diseases, cirrhosis and neuropsychiatric disorders; disinhibition and sexually transmitted diseases; unwanted pregnancy and complications in pregnancy including fetal distress;

and violence and suicide". Treatment and rehabilitation are essential components of demand reduction. They should be seen as a means to help persons overcome addiction and not a form of punishment. Research has indicated that treatment, carried out under proper conditions, does change behaviour. Treatment provides a necessary foundation for rehabilitation and community reintegration. The setting in which it occurs may be less important than the skills of persons involved, the processes used and the type of treatment. In planning to prevent relapse, many services are needed, including rehabilitation, community services and active follow-up. Successful programmes require qualified staff, constant management, adequate resources and the flexibility to adapt to changing circumstances.

Since resources for specialized assistance for persons with drug problems are often not available in many countries, existing primary health care settings and networks may have to be adapted to care for drug abusers. The majority of persons in rural areas have no easy access to specialized health care but primary health care networks can provide a contact point and a means of intervention. One expert has concluded that general health workers should receive training to deal with alcohol and drug problems, especially in such subjects as rapid assessment, counselling and crisis management of early phases of cases of substance abuse disorders.

Aggregate multicountry information on the costs of drug abuse is not available. In the United States, however, where this issue has been examined, drug abuse was found to impose a $44.1 billion dollar burden on the economy in 1985, with the projection of $58.3 billion for 1988. Calculations were based on the human capital approach, which is based on the value of productivity in terms of market earnings and imputed value for housekeeping services.

Drug abuse, compared to alcohol abuse and mental illness, was comparatively low in direct and indirect costs and high in other related costs, such as crime, motor vehicle crashes, administrative costs of related social welfare programmes and costs associated with the destruction of property by fire. This study's calculation of cost also included the value of productivity losses for victims of crime. Costs for men were twice that for women. The significantly higher costs for men reflect their higher prevalence as drug users, their greater labour force participation rates and their higher earnings relative to women. Estimates do not include costs of crack cocaine addiction and its devastating consequences because that problem emerged after this research was carried out in 1985. In the United Kingdom, the total identifiable costs associated, directly or indirectly, with drug abuse in 1988 were conservatively estimated at £1,821 million, with 80 per cent of this being the replacement value of stolen goods.

Investigation, legal and sentencing costs were other categories and preventive and medical costs were relatively minor. In Australia, researchers have examined alternative models to estimate costs, pointing out that any estimate may be misinterpreted. The researchers estimate that the annual avoidable tangible drug abuse costs for Australia for 1994 will be $AI 38 million. This amount is interpreted as indicating the potential benefit which could result from effective intervention programmes. Clearly, the preparation of social and economic cost estimates is becoming a priority. No comparative national estimates for the cost of care and treatment of substance abuse problems have been prepared. Most policy officials have little idea what the addictive disorders cost their countries or what they are spending on this group of problems.

In the United States, a study of hospital records shows a surprisingly high number of admissions and costs for substance-abuse-related treatment. This study found that in 1991, "there were 2.2 million tobacco, alcohol or drug-related Medicare admissions, which accounted for 20 per cent of all Medicare hospitalizations. Because these substance abuserelated cases tend to be more expensive to treat than the average hospital case, the amount actually paid by Medicare for substance abuse-related care was even higher, accounting for 23 per cent or nearly one-fourth of the total Medicare payments for hospital care. Substance abuse-related cases cost more to treat because they required almost 26 per cent more hospital staff and other resources than Medicare discharges that are unrelated to substance abuse". Furthermore, "Medicare spent over $13 billion of its $57 billion inpatient short-stay hospital expenditures on substance-abuse-related care. These amounts exceed the 1 out of 5 dollars spent in the Medicaid programme for substance abuse-related conditions". Although the magnitude of these figures is not typical of other countries, this same study found that "relying solely on diagnoses that explicitly mention alcohol or drugs on the medical record in order to measure the prevalence and cost of drugs and/or alcohol problems in hospitals grossly underestimates the full impact of substance abuse".

Cases where alcohol and drug treatment were the primary diagnoses represented less than 3 per cent of the substance-abuse total costs. The conclusion is that substance-abuse-related costs may be a serious but unrecognized drain on national income; it is often unrecognized because drugs or alcohol may not appear directly in diagnoses and classifications but may be major risk factors contributing to other diseases and costly social disorders. Paying for the costs of assistance to persons with drug problems raises many questions, including that of the role of the public and private sectors.

Many drug abusers are unable to pay the costs of care by themselves and have no insurance or other means to pay when health care is primarily provided by the private sector. Public policy should take into consideration two points. First, priority should be given to the most important aspects of the drug abuse problem, such as compulsive heroin or cocaine users' inability to pay for treatment. Involving them in public treatment programmes would reduce the demand for these drugs and allow supply reduction efforts to be more successful since the compulsive drug users consume far more drugs than experimenters.

Secondly, the issue of preventive care needs to be addressed. If preventive care systematically loses out to market forces, which are politically or commercially stronger, a government may need to intervene to ensure adequate support for prevention. The cost picture is made more complex by the nature of the existing health care system. Does a national or comprehensive health care system exist? If it does, are drug treatment services covered? A major policy issue is whether information on costs of the problem is sufficient to draw conclusions about resource allocation. In addition, estimates are needed about the costs of various alternative policy responses, including what the consequences would be if limited or no intervention takes place by authorities.

Allocation of scarce resources may be determined not only by costs associated with morbidity, mortality and associated social problems but also by other factors such as public perceptions of safety and security.

Although this discussion concerns the impact of illicit drugs, it should be borne in mind that many parts of the world lack adequate supplies of licit drugs, with neither essential medications nor access to basic health care.

Highlighting the abuse of dependence-producing drugs does not, however, diminish the magnitude of problems related to the unavailability of licit narcotics or psychotropics needed for treatment of health problems. Programmes to control the illicit use of drugs may be designed which support pharmaceutical control measures essential for distribution of licit drugs.

THE TREATMENT CENTRE FOR MEN

The Treatment Centre for Men was founded 18 years ago to address the critical gap faced by men facing addiction who need special assistance in their recovery. The Treatment Centre for Men is a private and exclusive nationally recognized and CARF accredited drug and alcohol treatment centre.

For men who need a more intensive and longer-term rehab programme to ensure long-term abstinence, the Extended Care Program offers more time to heal, learn, and adjust to a new life in recovery. This treatment programme of additional structure, focused attention, and safety is for chemically dependent and dually diagnosed men aged 18 and over. Every treatment plan at Michael's House is tailored for that individual's specific needs, begins with a 60-day stay, and can be extended according to each client's situation. Michael's House for Men is an intimate, tranquil, hacienda-style retreat that provides a beautiful, comfortable, and safe environment for recovery. The peaceful foothills of Mount San Jacinto, in Palm Springs, California, provide an ideal location for men seeking a private, single-sex drug and alcohol rehab environment where they may build a foundation of recovery in an atmosphere of complete safety and confidentiality.

RESIDENTIAL RETREAT AT MICHAEL'S HOUSE

The Residential Retreat Program offers men and women, age 18 and over, an integrated in-patient treatment programme serving persons with co-occurring conditions as well as drug and alcohol rehab. Our staff is specially trained in the The Foundations Treatment Model to address the complex needs of individuals with co-occurring disorders and addictions issues. The Retreat offers social setting Detox (detoxification services) and individualized integrated services for individuals with addictive and/or mental health conditions.

Treatment at Michael's House includes introduction to 12-step principles, daily group and individual therapy, and life skills classes. Residential programme participants enjoy delicious and nutritious food, an exercise weight room, meditation and quiet time, daily recreational opportunities, and other healthful and fun leisure activities. Nestled in the San Jacinto mountain range with breath taking views of the desert, the resort atmosphere offers safety and privacy while going through the detoxification process as well as beginning to address issues surrounding alcoholism, drug addiction, and co-occurring disorders.

ALCOHOL REHAB

Effective alcohol rehabilitation programmes provide a variety of services aimed at meeting the treatment goals and needs of the people they serve. At

Michael's House, you or your loved one determines the pace for alcohol rehabilitation according to your (or your loved one's) readiness to recover or change. Alcohol rehab at Michael's House includes:

Development of relapse prevention skills, education about alcoholism, as well as information about other conditions that might be present, introduction to 12-Step principles, and identification of relapse triggers. Evaluation for medication treatments to control cravings or reduce withdrawal symptoms is recognized as a viable option and if a mental health condition is also present, medications might also be necessary to treat that condition.

Many alcohol rehab programmes have historically strictly provided alcohol rehab without attention to other mental issues. However, given the impact of addiction on other life issues, it is no surprise that mental health complications are very common among those who participate in alcohol rehab programmes. In fact, more than 44% of alcoholics have mental health complications prior to the onset of alcohol dependence and many others develop mood-related complications, such as depression and dysthymia, after the onset of the addiction.

We now know the importance of alcohol rehab centres to incorporate mental health treatments in addition to alcohol rehab services and at Michael's House we know how to treat these co-occurring disorders.

Bibliography

Andrew, N.: *Foundations of Nanomechanics: from Solid-state Theory to Device Applications,* Berlin, New York, 2003.

Attebery, B.: *Nanoculture: Implications of the New Technoscience,* Bristol, Intellect Books, 2004.

Charles, P., and Frank J. Owens: *Introduction to Nanotechnology,* Hoboken, J. Wiley, 2003.

Credi, A.: *Molecular Devices and Machines: a Journey into the Nano World,* Weinheim, Wiley-VCH, 2003.

Daniel Ratner: *Nanotechnology: a Gentle Introduction to the Next Big Idea,* Upper Saddle River, Prentice Hall, 2003.

Drexler, K. Eric: *Engines of Creation: The Coming Era of Nanotechnology,* New York, Anchor Books, 1986.

Frank J. Owens: *Introduction to Nanotechnology,* Hoboken, J. Wiley, 2003.

Fukuyama F.: *Our Posthuman Future: Consequences of the Biotechnology Revolution,* NewYork: Farrar, Straus and Giroux, 2002.

Fumento, Michael: *Bioevolution: How Biotechnology is Changing Our World,* San Francisco, California: Encounter Books, 2003.

Gaskell, G: *Biotechnology - the Making of a Global Controversy,* Cambridge, Cambridge University Press, 2002.

Gregory, L.: *Nanotechnology,* New York, Springer, 1999.

Harris J.: *Wonderwoman & Superman: the Ethics of Human Biotechnology,* Oxford, Oxford University Press, 1992.

Hayles, N.K. : *Nanoculture: Implications of the New Technoscience,* Bristol, Intellect Books, 2004.

Hessenbruch, A.: *Nanotechnology and the Negotiation of Novelty,* Amsterdam, IOS Press, 2004.

Katz, E., R. Lovel, W. Mee and F. Solomon: *Citizens' Panel on Nanotechnology: Report to Participants,* Melbourne, CSIRO Minerals, 2005.

Kurzweil, Ray: *The Age of Spiritual Machines,* New York, Penguin Books, 1999.

Lewis, J.: *Prospects in Nanotechnology: Toward Molecular Manufacturing,* New York, John Wiley & Sons, 1995.

Mark, A., and Daniel Ratner: *Nanotechnology: a Gentle Introduction to the Next Big Idea,* Upper Saddle River, Prentice Hall, 2003.

Meyer, M.: *Socio-economic Research on Nanoscale Science and Technology: A European Overview and Illustration,* Dordrecht, Kluwer, 2001.

Moravec, Hans: *Mind Children: The Future of Robot and Human Intelligence,* Cambridge, Harvard University Press, 1988.

Moravec, Hans: *Mind Children: The Future of Robot and Human Intelligence,* Cambridge, Harvard University Press, 1988.

Nigel, M. De S. Cameron: *Human Dignity in the Biotech Century: A Christian Vision for Public Policy,* Downers Grove, InterVarsity Press, 2004.

Norio Taniguchi: *Nanotechnology: Integrated Processing Systems for Ultra-precision and Ultra-fine Products,* New York, Oxford University Press, 1996.

Orth, R. N.: *Nanometer Scale Antibody Patterning for Directed cell Immobilization and Stimulation,* Ithaca, Cornell University, 2002.

Owens, J.: *Introduction to Nanotechnology,* Hoboken, J. Wiley, 2003.

Parens, Erik: *Enhancing Human Traits: Ethical and Social Implications,* Washington, D.C., Georgetown University Press, 1998.

Paul, S.: *Beyond Humanity: Cyber Evolution and Future Minds,* Roackland, Charles River Media, 1996.

Postman, Neil: *Technopoly: The Surrender of Culture to Technology,* New York, Vintage Books, 1992.

Pressman, J.: *Nano Narrative: A Parable from Electronic Literature,* Bristol, Intellect Books, 2004.

Ratner, D.: *Nanotechnology: a Gentle Introduction to the Next Big Idea,* Upper Saddle River, Prentice Hall, 2003.

Richard, Hewlett: *A Policy Framework for Developing a National Nanotechnology Program,* Blacksburg, University Libraries, 1998.

Rietman, Ed.: *Molecular Engineering of Nanosystems,* New York, Springer, 2001.

Roobeek, A: *The Biotechnology Revolution?,* Oxford, Blackwell, 1995.

Rosalyn, W. : *Encyclopedia of Science, Technology and Ethics,* Detroit, Thomson-Gale, 2005.

Sarewitz, D.: *Nanotechnology and Societal Transformation,* Dordrecht, Kluwer, 2001.

Schummer, J.: *Interdisciplinary Issues in Nanoscale Research,* Amsterdam: IOS Press, 2004.

Seeman, N.: *DNA Nanotechnology for Massive Information Storage,* New York, New York University, 2001.

Smith, H. A.: *Nanotechnology Infrared Optics for Astronomy Missions,* Washington, National Aeronautics and Space Administration, 2002.

Srivastava, D.: *Nanotechnology based Materials and Devices for Health Care,* Moffett Field, Computer Sciences Corp., 2002.

Stephen M. Goodnick: *Transport in Nanostructures,* Cambridge, Cambridge University Press, 1997.

Suchman, M.: *Envisioning Life on the Nano-Frontier,* Dordrecht, Kluwer, 2001.

Tenner, E.: *Nanotechnology and Unintended Consequences,* , Dordrecht, Kluwer, 2001.

Tomellini, R.: *Nanotechnology: Revolutionary Opportunities and Societal Implications, Workshop, Lecce,* Luxemburg: Office for Official Publications of the European Communities, 2002.

Weil, V.: *Ethical Issues in Nanotechnology,* Dordrecht, Kluwer, 2001.

Index

M

N

O

P

R

S

T

V

❑❑❑